Guava as medicine

Guava as medicine

A safe and cheap form of Food Therapy

INGFRIED HOBERT, M.D.
HARALD W. TIETZE

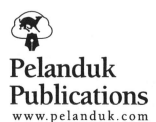

Pelanduk
Publications
www.pelanduk.com

IMPORTANT LEGAL NOTICE
This publication seeks to demonstrate the beneficial application of herbs for various disorders of the human body. However, it must be stressed that the contents of this book are in no way a substitute for personal supervision by qualified professional medical personnel. The contents of this publication are solely the opinions of the authors and people with health problems should consult their physicians.

Published in 2001 by
Pelanduk Publications (M) Sdn Bhd
(Co. No. 113307-W)
12 Jalan SS13/3E
Subang Jaya Industrial Estate
47500 Subang Jaya
Selangor Darul Ehsan, Malaysia

Address all correspondence to
Pelanduk Publications (M) Sdn Bhd
P.O. Box 8265, 46785 Kelana Jaya
Selangor Darul Ehsan, Malaysia

Visit our website at *www.pelanduk.com*
e-mail: *mypp@tm.net.my*

Copyright © 1998 Harald W. Tietze
All rights reserved. No part of this book may be reproduced in any form or by any means without prior permission from the copyright holder. Published by arrangement with Harald W. Tietze Publishing Pty Ltd, Australia.

ISBN 967-978-779-6

Printed by
Cetakmurni Sdn Bhd

"And God said: Behold, I have given you every herb bearing seed, which is upon the face of all the earth, and every tree, in which is the fruit of a tree yielding seed; to you it shall be for meat." (1. Moses 1, 29)

"Your food should be your medicine and your medicine should be your food" (Hippokrates)

"Humans are the only living creatures on earth eating food altered and devalued by heat" (Professor Dr Kollath)

Contents

Acknowledgement
Preface

Guava—A Tropical Plant with Incredible Healing Power	1
The History and Origin of the Guava	1
The Different Names of the Guava	2
The Relatives of the Guava	3
The Most Known Varieties	3
Strawberry Guava	3
Cherry Guava	4
When is a Guava not a Guava	4
Pineapple Guava or Feijoa	4
The Australian Guava	5
Cultivation of the Guava	6
The Leaves	9
The Flowers	9
The Fruits	10
The Most Known Commercial Varieties	11
Guava as an Indoor Plant	14
As Medicinal Plant, only the *Psidium guava* should be grown	14
Guava for the Pleasure of the Taste Buds	17
Keeping Healthy and Fit	18
Guava Recipes	19

Guava as Medicine	25
Guava–A Healing Remedy Worldwide	26
Science Discovered the Healing Power of Guava	28
Composition and Operation	33
Fruits	33
Leaves	33
How to Make and Use Your Own Guava Medicine	34
Conservation of Guava	34
Juice	35
Drying	35
Careful Drying but Without Microwave	36
Seeds	37
Wine	38
Beer	38
The Best Preservation: Lactic Acid Fermentation	38
Guave Sauer-Herb Fermentation	40
Fermentation with the Kombucha Culture	41
Guava-Papaya-Concentrate	42
A Particularly Good Combinations: Guave-Papaya-Concentrate	43
Guava Preparations	44
Why Do Bees Love Guava Leaves?	46
Homeopathic Guava	53
How to Make Homeopathic Guava Medicine	55
Guava Flower Essence	57
The Stepanovs Method	58
Advantages of the Stepanovs Method	59
Application of the Guava flower Essence	60

Applications of Guava of A–Z	60
Guava for Health and Beauty	81
Guava Skin Care	81
Guava Body Care	84
Guava Foot Care	88
Other Uses of Guava	90
Wood for Smoking for the Barbecue	90
Tanning of Leather	90
Wood Processing	90
Dyeing	91
Washing After Burial	91
Dental Hygiene	91
Practical Hints for Better Health and Vigour	91
The Way to Freedom	93
Final Remark from Harald	94
Bibliography	*98*
References	*101*

Acknowledgement

Special thanks to all our friends from 22 countries, who helped with information for this book. Particular thanks go to the Illawarra Philipino Womens Group from Wollongong, Australia, who went to a lot of trouble, to collected from their members the traditional uses of guava to share with others for better health. A particular thanks to our women Juta and Astrid for their support and their patience during our work on the desk after midnight or long before sunrise.

> *"Harald Tietze's modesty would not permit him to reveal how popular his health books are, but I know for a fact one of his most popular book has been published in more than a dozen languages! In fact I would not be surprised if he isn't the most published author in the world today in home and natural health remedies.*
>
> *The whole field of plant medicine has taken a quantum leap in the last decade, and Harald's latest book* Guava, Medicine for Modern Diseases *co-authored with Ingfried Hobert, M.D. is a milestone in this development.*
>
> *Harald draws upon his past successful health publications to bring to bear knowledge on the value of Guava in health. His most popular book on Kombucha (referred to above) provides the method to brew Guava vinegar (p.48).*
>
> *I heartily recommend this great authors latest book".*
>
> Dr William L. Mayo

Preface

"Logical thinking brings us no real wisdom of the empirical world, all knowledge of reality begins and ends with one's own experience".
— Albert Einstein

Curiously, knowing that there is still so much between heaven and earth that we do not yet know, and that cannot be proven with rational scientific laws, searching nowadays sends us more deeply, over the horizon of our own dinner plates, around the world. Inspired by the hope of discovering new ways, or to see new perspectives, we began our research with natives who still live their same lifestyle as they have done throughout history and we studied how they maintain health and fight diseases.

It is our aim to find in the traditional ceremonies of old cultures the answers to many questions, and understand their mysterious energies, which are necessary to maintain our existence.

Native Schamans medicine still existing today, have known since primeval times about the mysterious powers controlling life–both in the jungle and cities alike.

Shamanism is not only the oldest way of healing for mankind, it proves today that it is mentally and emotionally an adventure through which we are to discover a new reality and scoop power for health, against disease and death and to enjoy life.

The search for the source of health and vigour can only begin in nature itself. Nature has created itself from itself in such a perfect and abundant way, that it quickly becomes clear that the treasure of nature is so rich, that it has an answer for every question and a herb for every illness.

There are in the fruitful jungle, plants with extraordinary healing powers, whose incredible effects were discovered and studied only in recent times. One such plant is the guava with its wonderful nutritional and healing power.

Guava has given people health and vigour for thousands of years. Today, guava is planted around the world in tropical areas.

Guava is today's treasure worldwide as medicinal plants with a wide spectrum of healing benefits. The nutritional value and the multitude of particular ingredients makes guava an outstanding healing plant.

Guava was used throughout history by many cultures. The knowledge about its medicinal uses has been built up from observations (without scientific double-blind studies) in the countries of origin like South and Middle America but also in other tropical countries around the world and is a guarantee for the efficiency of guava. How small and insignificant are the so-called high scientific studies of today, carried out with only a few hundred people over a few months or years.

Even in modern time when we know so much and learn so much about proper nourishment, we still make many dietary mistakes. The fact that two-thirds of all our diseases in western society is caused by poor nourishment should trigger some thinking process most of us. Every second bed in our hospitals is filled with a patient eating him/herself to this undesired but avoidable condition.

It is very difficult for every individual to protect themselves against diseases caused by poor nutrition.

Unfortunately today we are exposed to a multitude of poisonous substances in our food. Our body has to tolerate them whether it wants to or not. In the long-term, with a build-up of stress factors influencing our lives, our defence system collapses and were ending up in hospital or worse.

One only has to think about dyes, preservatives, synthetic aroma, taste enhancers and many other industrial reconditioning and manufacturing processes, and last but not least, the *microwaving* of food in kitchens.

The question is essential, how much natural food are we taking daily and how much for health and life-living natural energy is still in our daily food.

It seems to become very clear that humans cannot live from artificial products only. The need for so-called vitality food, natural plants including herbs, which the body needs to be healthy and vital becomes clear.

It was believed that it is possible to manufacture everything artificially in a laboratory, but since the dissemination of the genetic manipulated tomatoes, the so-called Holland-tomato, everyone found out for themselves how something like this tastes and even more what there is in it and what it does to us in the long-term.

To all the above, one has to consider that almost every day new artificial ingredients and trace minerals are discovered which nobody knew of before.

It is therefore obvious, that we must begin to take our life in our hands and personally search for a food in which there is at the same time medicine. We have to start to learn to think for ourselves.

Guava—A Tropical Plant with Incredible Healing Power

The History and Origin of the Guava

There are many varieties of guava. This book tells in the first line about the use of the most potent guava, the *Psidium guajava*, for nutrition and healing

Guava belongs to the family of the Myrtaceae, the Family that most common Australian trees such as Tea-tree and the Eucalyptus belong to.

In many countries guava belongs among the most important plants of the natives. One example is Peru where guava was cultivated, probably for thousands of years. In archaeological excavations in Peru guava seeds along with beans, corn and other seeds were found, which proves that guavas were planted thousands of years ago, in the earliest agriculture.

Nowadays guava is cultivated around the world in all tropical countries. Guava is very easy to grow and tolerates both very moist soil as well as dry locations. Guava tolerates very high temperatures and survives temporarily flooding without problems. In areas where there is a cool season, the trees carry more fruit and have fewer diseases.

Guava grows relatively quickly 3–10m high, upright and with a hard wood trunk.

In some countries guavas are spreading undesirably fast. The birds love the fruit and carry the seeds, together with fertiliser, in the most remote areas. But also pigs, cattle and horses love the fruit and likewise spread the seeds.

The strawberry guava is in some countries like Hawaii, a weed which spreads very fast and competes with the native plants.

The Different Names of the Guava

Guajava is the original name of the Tupi—Indians, from tropical America. Here names such as Goiaba, Guayaba, Guayabas, Kuava, Kuyabas, where derived.

In some books it is mentioned that Guava is the original name from the Incas and Mayas.

When I asked friends from Mexico and Peru about Guava, they didn't know anything about this plant. After giving a more detailed description of guava and its uses, they said it must be the guajava, which, considering the Latin name explains it.

In Mexico it is called Xalxocotl. From this the Portuguese derived the word Peer (pear). This name was spread then in the colonies, with derivatives such as Perakka, Perala, Petokal, Peyara, Piyara.

Here are some of the most frequently used names for guava in alphabetical sequence:

Abas, Amarood, Amrud, Araca, Batu, Bayawas, Bayabas, Biyawas, Enandi, Guayaba, Dipajava, Djamboe, Djambu, Fan Shi Liu, Farang, Goavier, Goiaba,

Gouyava, Goyavier, Guyaaba, Guayabo, Guayaba, Guayabas, Guyava, Guyavus, Jambu, Jamphal, Jamrukh, Jamu, Kayawase, Klutuk, Kowayas, Koyabas, Koyabasa, Kuava, Kuyabas, Malacka Pela, Mapun, Melakut, Perakka, Perala, Petokal, Peyara, Pichi, Piyara, Posh, Tokal, Sapari, Waiawi, Wuyamas, Xalxocotl.

The Relatives of the Guava

Altogether there are about 150 guavas. Most of them have, according to reports, no value in the fruits and leaves.

The Most Known Varieties

Strawberry Guava, or Cattley Guava (*Psidium cattleianum*). Also called Guisaro or Brazilian guava (*Psidium guinense*) or as it is called in Brazil the ula-ula or waiawi.

This guava is planted in Gardens not only because of the fruit but also as ornamental tree or bush or as an evergreen hedge.

Strawberry Guava has leathery dark green leaves up to 6m long. The red round fruit is 2–3cm in size. The birds love strawberry guava and one can only harvest fruit if the entire bush is covered with a net, long before the berries become ripe.

From the berries a delicious jelly and jam can be made.

An excellent wine is also made from the berries.

Strawberry guava is a major problem in Hawaii, where it was cultivated at the turn of the century. The strawberry guava loves the climate and soil on the dream island so much, that it became one of the most unpopular weeds in Hawaii, spreading even in the jungle. Colder temperatures do not harm the strawberry guava. It can be planted in cool areas without difficulties.

Cherry Guava (*Psidium cattleianum littorale*) is one closely related to the red strawberry guava having yellow, often somewhat orange fruit. The bush has more and denser branches. The fruits are mostly larger than the fruits of the strawberry guava.

When is a Guava not a Guava

It is always very difficult if two totally different things have the same name. Similar plants have sometimes been called the same name although it deals with a totally different plant, which are not even related like the following.

Pineapple guava or **Feijoa** (*Feijoa sellowina*) originates in South America and adopts quite well also in cooler zones as in Argentina. Pineapple guava is an evergreen bush with dark green leaves. Long droughts, which are common in some areas, do not harm Pineapple guava. Pineapple guava has very attractive, white or red blossoms and is therefore planted in cooler climates as a fruit bearing ornamental bush.

I have one in my garden and was astonished one day, to find fruit under the bush which I thought did not bear fruits. I tasted the pineapple guava which was not yet ripe. It has a terrible taste drawing my whole face together. A friend, whom I questioned for advice whether the fruit may be poisonous, told me that the fruits have to be fully ripe.

Pineapple guavas must be fully ripe to taste well. There are only about 2 days between being fully ripe and starting to rot! The fruit flies love the Pineapples guavas very much.

The fruit are hidden under the branches and leaves which have the same colour. As the name says, pineapples guavas taste like pineapples, or fruit salad. Pineapple guava is not offered in green grocery shops since they do not keep long and attract fruit flies.

Australian Guava (*Eupomatia laurina*) is for botanists a very interesting tree, because it is one of the most primitive blooming plants still existing. This guava adjusts to different locations very well. It is found along the east coast of Australia, from the tropical north in Queensland down to the cool south in Victoria. The Aborigines call it Bolwarra which was part of their diet.

The leaves of this native guava are attractive dark green, the blossoms of creamy colour. The fruits are the size of the common fig with many seeds in the clear flesh. The fruits are 2–3cm long and ripen in the winter. If they are ripe, they become soft and yellowish-green. The taste is pleasant, aromatic and sweet and reminds one of the tastes of the guava. That is the reason it got the misleading name.

Cultivation of Guava

Modern tropical agriculture, which has to produce cheaply, is forced, to use chemicals, even if these have poor effects for the consumer. The difference to agriculture in countries with cold winters and hard frost is that fungal diseases and vermin pests can reproduce in tropical areas all-year "optimally", while the frost in countries with a strong winter helps to control plant diseases.

Guava is fortunately a very robust tree. The main problem is the fruit fly and the birds, which love the fruit even if it draws peoples' mouths or even the entire face together.

Young trees cannot tolerate frost, even low temperatures close to freezing point can damage a young Guava tree. Larger trees survive frosts to minus 6°C for some hours, which can happen sometimes inland and at higher altitudes before sunrise. It is then possible that the tree loses its leaves but they will grow back fast.

Guavas have flat roots and can be planted in big containers or large flowerpots in the green house or even as an indoor plant. More on this in the chapter "Guava as an Indoor Plant."

Guava requires a rainfall of 1000–2000mm per year. The vegetation temperature is between 20°C and 30°C. Guavas grow at an altitude of 2100m above sea level.

The quality of the fruit is not good if the humidity is too high or if there is not enough rain. The best fruit quality as regards to taste is when the harvest of the ripe fruit is at the beginning of the dry season.

To produce good quality fruit, plantations are not irrigated during that time.

Fruit rot and parasites can become a problem in tropical plantations during the rainy season. In more moderate zones one has none of these difficulties.

In commercial production one distinguishes the varieties of fruits for the consumer markets, fruits to produce juice or puree and fruits which suit for both.

Immature fruit smell unpleasant but ripe guavas smell very pleasant. They can sometimes look unsightly, but taste good.

Green guavas have a higher healing potential than ripe fruit. The natives take them for diarrhoea and other complaints. The guava loves soil with high nutrients, with a high percentage of organic matter. Nevertheless it tolerates almost all types of soil but prefers a soil pH of 5–7. Guava tolerates limited flooding e.g. water locking but is sensitive against high levels of salt in the soil.

Grafting is not simple but it is very easy to make new plants by layering from branches, suckers or from the root.

Guavas can be grown from seeds, which should come from preferably large, pleasant tasting fruits. Plants grown from seeds bear first fruits after 4–5 years. Plants grown from cuttings already begin to carry fruits after 2 and at the latest 3 years.

Cuttings are taken from trees which carry especially good crops. At the age of 8 years the trees deliver good crops and produce up to an age of 30 years.

The fruit needs 100–150 days depending on rains and temperature from the blossom to the ripe fruit.

One calculates at 40kg fruit per year per mature tree in plantations.

The tree tolerates heavy pruning, however it must be considered that the fruit develops only at the young branches. The removal of old and young wood must be well balanced.

Since Guavas carry a lot of fruit it is recommended that to produce large fruit, one must thin out when small or prune back a balanced amount of the young fruit bearing branches. This method has the further advantage, that fewer branches break under the load of the fruit and the tree produces better new fruit throughout the whole year

A guava tree is very decorative, needs little or no maintenance, produces much fruit and is a medicine plant of high value. A guava tree should be in every garden where the climate allows it.

The Leaves

The leaves develop the whole year through. They are 10–15cm long, bright green, oblong-oval and leathery. On the underside there are clearly raised veins. The leaves are used in many countries as effective medicine against many health problems. They are also sometimes called *Djamboe*.

It is always good to have a guava tree in the garden to have medicine ready if needed like chewing leaves against tooth ache. It is always good to have leaves from your own trees as in commercial plantations trees are sometimes sprayed with chemicals to cause part of their fruit and leaves to drop in order to produce bigger fruits.

When purchasing tea one should make sure that it comes from biological production.

The Flowers

The little white fragrant blossoms develop at the young branches in tropical climates all the year, if there are no rains or extreme temperatures to influence this. In cool areas they bloom only twice per year. For example they bloom in the north of India according to rainfall two to three times annually and in the south always three times. Only once a year in cooler climate.

Two or three blossoms, each about 2.5–3cm long, develop in the leave axils.

Guava does not need another guava tree at close proximity for pollination. However the fruits develop better, particularly if seeds are taken for germination or if the bees mix pollen of other guavas, Flower essences can be made from the fresh blossoms without cutting them using the *Stepanovs Method*.

The Fruits

There are various shapes of fruit like pears, lemons or apples, therefore it is called pears-, apple- or lemons-guava. They become 4–10cm long and weigh between 100 and 450gm.

Guava fruit are very high in vitamin C, but also in vitamins A and B.

There are many varieties of guavas from white fruit flesh to red. Fruit with white flesh are sweeter than the pink fruit, which tastes of acid or sour. In optimal climates, the guava tree bears fruit the whole year-round. In cooler zones, fruits are harvested only in the warmer months. The size of the fruits fluctuates with the seasons.

For fresh fruit storage it is important to know that tropical fruit cannot ripen in the refrigerator. Immature picked fruit will never unfold their full aroma. The immature fruit is harvested for medicinal purposes. For best taste take the fruit direct from the tree when fully ripe. Immature guavas are harvested for transport in far countries. These must ripen then at room temperature, so that aroma can develop as well as possible. Ripe fruit can be stored in the refrigerator. Similarly like some other tropical fruit, such as the mango, immature guavas have an unpleasant smell.

The Most Known Commercial Varieties

Beaumont is a medium-sized to large fruit, with a weight up to 240gm. The flesh is light red, has many seeds and tastes mildly acidic. The tree produces many fruit.

Detwiler is a medium-sized, round fruit, with a diameter of about 7cm. The skin is greenish-yellow; the flesh yellow to orange, has many seeds and tastes relatively sweet, with a good aroma. The tree produces many fruit.

Hong Kong Pink is a medium-sized round fruit with a weight of 189–240gm. The flesh is pink/red, has little seeds and tastes relatively acid-sweet, with a good aroma. The tree produces many fruit.

Mexican Cream is a small to medium-sized round fruit. The skin is yellowish with red marks. The flesh is creamy-white, has little soft seeds and tastes very sweet. The tree grows upright.

Red Indian is a medium-sized to large, round fruit. The green skin has reddish spots. The flesh is of good quality, has many small seeds, is red and tastes sweet. It is a good fruit for the market.

Ruby X This hybrid variety was bred in Florida, USA. The small round fruit is greenish-yellow. The flesh has relatively little seeds, is red-orange and tastes excellent. It is a bushy tree.

Sweet White Indonesian is one of the largest varieties with round fruits, which can reach 10cm or more in the diameter. They are yellowish; the robust flesh is sweet and tastes very good. The tree increases very quickly and bears good crops.

White Indian The 5–7cm round fruit, has a robust, white flesh with little seeds. The taste is outstanding and spicy. The tree produces only small fruit.

White Seedless is a variety, as the name says with no seeds. The flesh is, as that from the White India, white.

Worldwide demand for guava is increasing, particularly for the delightful juice.

The world production is approximately 500,000 tons. India is the biggest producer, with an annual production of 165,000 tons of guava or Peyara as it is called there. Further major exporting countries are South Africa, Brazil, Thailand and Mexico.

The seeds in the ripe fruit are hard but one can remove them easily. Similar to figs, the seeds are eaten with the soft fruit flesh.

There are also guavas without kernels, which are grown in large plantations in India. Other varieties may have 100 to over 500 seeds. It is more enjoyable to eat a fruit with many little seeds than a fruit with only a few seeds but big seeds.

The seeds germinate very easily within 2–3 weeks under optimal conditions. To produce new trees, the seeds are taken from especially large, pleasant tasting fruit.

Dry seeds contain about 14% oil and 15% protein.

The bark is relatively smooth, light brown to reddish brown, sometimes moss green. Similar to Eucalyptus trees, the bark comes off in shreds.

In poor countries the dried bark is sold sometimes as cinnamon, after it is treated with cinnamon oil.

One distinguishes the bark for medicinal purposes between the internal bark and the outer bark. The internal bark is soft and clean and is therefore preferred to treat inflamed skin or injuries.

The root system is shallow and wide spreading around the tree to collect every drop of rain. Relatively few roots are going deep in the ground. Plants grown from root cuttings usually do not have many root going deep in the ground. These trees are very susceptible to strong storms.

In light soils, the roots are susceptible to Nematodes (*Meloidogyne* sp.). The bark of the roots, as well as young roots, like the bark of the stem is used medicinally.

Guava as an Indoor Plant

Not everyone would like to live in the tropics and not everyone who wants to live in the tropics lives there, but everyone can grow guava. It grows best in the tropics with the average temperature ranging from 24°C–25°C. Guava also tolerates a soil pH of 4.3–8 but the plant can grow with readings above or below this value. The ideal soil pH is 6. The plant needs a well-drained soil as like the roots of the Papaya, will rot if the soil is water logged for too long. The tree likes the sun, and frost will kill it. Guava grows quite well in containers and is suitable as an indoor plant occasionally taken outdoors in spring.

The guava tree is fairly easy to grow and with a little bit of feeling for this tropical plant everyone can grow guava at home and use the sprouts as a healthy ingredient in salads or the leaves as medicinal tea.

As Medicinal Plant, only the *Psidium guajava* should be grown

Seeds To buy seeds one need not go to a nursery. Guava seeds are offered in grocery stores in a very neat packaging—the fruit. In the tropics insects take care of the cleaning and if the seed is eaten by birds when they eat the flesh of the fruit, the digestion of the birds takes care of both the cleaning of the seeds and the fresh fertiliser required for faster growth when they are both dropped together! It is best to use fresh seeds within one or two weeks of purchase, since the germination rate is affected by storage. For long-term storage the seed has to be dried at a maximum of 45°C and then stored in airtight containers on a cool spot. Under optimal storage conditions a good germination rate after one year is reported. For commercial growing the seeds are treated with chemicals against fungal diseases.

Clean seeds germinate within 2–3 weeks at optimal temperatures of 26°C high humidity. If the temperature is too low the seeds will rot.

Never throw seeds away. Dry the seeds or germinate all the seeds, mainly to produce guava sprouts and young leaves.

Germinating Dried Seeds Dried seeds are soaked for two days in water. The water is changed twice a day. The best time to put the seeds in containers is late winter. The plants can then develop indoors and be planted out in the open in spring. Of course you should not place the plants directly into bright sunlight, they must first be hardened in the shade.

The seeds are usually germinated in shallow containers and when the little plants develop two or three true leaves they are then separated. These are then planted 5–8cm apart or in bigger containers. When the plants are 20–30cm high they are planted into their permanent spot or in the final container. For indoor plants the final container should be 50–60cm high to give the roots around ½m of soil. This container can be placed into a water basin with water 5cm deep which makes daily watering unnecessary.

Instead of using a shallow germination container I fill a clear plastic container (with a clear lid) available in supermarkets. The container is about two feet long and one foot wide and one foot deep. I fill it to a depth of 20cm with potting mix and put enough water in it so that it stands 1–2cm from the bottom. The water is enriched with organic fertiliser. Since I live in the southern part of Australia, which is not really hot enough I place the container on a Kombucha heating panel which guarantees me good germination and plant growth.

The warm bottom of the container causes water to evaporate and condense on the lid. In this way the plants in the early stages of germination are constantly watered.

This unit is extremely cheap, effective and makes an ideal microclimate for the tropical plant.

When the plants are 10cm high the lid is taken off so that the plants can develop properly. The water level has to be checked every few days. With a clear container it is very easy, since you see the water level through the clear plastic. With non-clear plastic containers it is simple to check the water level by putting a little pipe in one corner and one can check very easily if there is still water on the bottom. This container is very effective for growing Guava sprouts between 20 and 30cm high. Since one does not need hundreds of Guava trees the sprouts are taken out. The whole plant, with the roots attached, is washed and used in salads like vegetables, or blended in a kitchen mixer along with other fruit juices to make a healthy drink.

If the sprouts are used for growing trees they are transferred when they are 20cm high and planted in a large container as described before. Since guava is a tree which grows up to very high outdoors, it is advisable to cut off the top of the tree when it is about 1–1½ m high. The tree will then develop more branches and will not grow straight up to the ceiling of the room. Guava is a good-looking exotic indoor plant and it is best placed in a sunny position.

Guava for the Pleasure of the Taste Buds

Our body is daily confronted with big loads of unnatural food. On one hand our digestion must deal everyday with poisonous substances which have to be separated and expelled in the shortest time possible. On the other hand our body in western societies is overloaded with "too much" food which has to be digested, separated utilised and so on. Our body has to filter out the qualitatively valuable components which are needed for efficient metabolism to maintain health.

Keeping Healthy and Fit

1. Avoid poisonous substances in your food i.e. avoid eating industrially or chemically altered foods.
2. Take time, i.e. eat slowly and chew well.
3. Eat pure living natural food, i.e. consume harvested natural products as fresh as possible in the form of fruit, salad and vegetables.
4. Consume "food medicine" in addition, i.e., nourish the body with plants which one knows, have a health giving effect, like fresh dandelion, papaya, guava.
5. Do not eat unnecessarily.

Guava is one of many fruit, which displays a very high capacity of vital components and is treasured in many countries of this earth as an excellent medicinal plant. While it is best to all fruit when it is ripe, for healing purposes guava is used green.

Only fully ripe guavas are pleasure for the taste buds and even better, when they are coming fresh from the tree.

As remedies, the immature fruit is essentially better. Fruits, which are harvested green for long transport to colder areas, have therefore a higher medicinal value. One does not have to live in the tropics, to be able to buy fresh tropical medicine.

Since the guava leaves, the bark and the roots have high medicinal value it is very beneficial to have a guava tree in the garden or as an indoor plant.

From every part of the plant one can make wonderful preparations in a home environment.

Guava Recipes

Guava Juice

The stems are removed and the fruit is washed, cut in small slices, weighed and put into a saucepan. Per 1kg fruit 1 litre of water is added. It is boiled shortly and then simmered for 20 minutes. After the juice has cooled down, it is sieved through a cheesecloth. One cup of sugar, one teaspoon of tartaric acid is added per two cups of juice. The juice is then heated again and filled in bottles, which are locked immediately

Guava Cream

> 1kg (can or glass) of guava fruit with juice
> 1 cup sweetened condensed milk
> 1 tablespoon gelatine dissolved in ¼ cup cold water
> 2 eggs
> 1 pinch salt

Cook the guava. Separate the juice and add so much water to fill two cups

Heat the juice again, remove it from the stove and add the gelatine stir allow to cool down.

Beat the white egg with a pinch of salt until stiff. Gently fold it into the above mixture when it is about to set. It is then poured into a mould and refrigerated.

Serve with custard, made from the egg yolk.

Guava soup

In China a soup is prepared from the fruit and leaves, which is used in first line for diabetics. Other ingredients are added as well. The leaves are not eaten with the soup since they are too tough.

Guava Jam

The fruits are peeled and cut into slices and placed into a pot.

Water is added, to just cover the fruit. The fruits are cooked until tender. Let cool down and add to each kg fruit with water 1kg sugar. Heat again slowly until the sugar has dissolved and then cook for further 30 minutes until the mass is firm and fill the prepared glasses.

Guava Jelly

1kg fine sliced Guava
1.2kg sugar
¼ cup of lemon juice

Both ends of the Guavas are cut and than cut in fine slices. Double as much water as fruit is put into a pot. Simmer for 40 minutes. As soon as it is cool enough, strain through a cheesecloth. This juice is placed back into the pot. The sugar and lemon juice is added and cooked rapidly to the setting point and filled into the prepared jars.

After cooling down a small nip of rum is added, not only to improve the taste but also to prevent mould.

The remaining pulp may be used for Guava cheese.

Guava Cheeses

> 1kg Guava pulp (left over from making jelly)
> 1kg sugar
> 1 tablespoon butter
> 1 teaspoon salt
> ¼ Cup of lemon juice

The pulp is cooked with the sugar and salt until it begins to jelly, when the lemon juice is added. Continue boiling until it starts to come away from the wall of the pot. The mixture should have a temperature of 115°C. Butter is now added. Stir well, and remove from the stove. The mixture is poured on a greased plate and left to cool. After cooling down it is cut into cubes and stored in an airtight container.

Guava Snack

This recipe originates from Africa.

Guavas are cooked until soft. The seeds are removed and the pulp is further cooked. Stir at intervals until thick.

A little water is added if necessary.

The mass is poured thinly on a glass plate and left to dry in the sun for 2 or 3 days. It is then cut into strips and stored in airtight containers. This dried fruit snack keeps well and is healthy.

Guava Nectar

> 500g small chopped guavas
> 200g sugars
> ¼ litres of water
> 125ml lemon juice

The Guavas are cooked with the water and the sugar until tender. Lemon juice is mixed to the pulp. The seeds are removed by straining it through a cheesecloth.

For nectar, the pulp is diluted with water in a ratio 1:2.5.

The pulp may also be frozen in cubes for later use for tasty drinks, to make jelly or pudding.

Guava Spice Cake

> 3½ cups guava pulp
> 2 eggs

¾ cup skim milk powder
½ cup maple syrup
1 teaspoon grated orange skin
1 teaspoon cinnamon
1 knife tip ground macon
1 knife tip ground ginger
thin carambola slices
butter-whipped cream to decorate.

Guava, eggs, milk powder, maple syrup and spices are mixed together with a kitchen mixer and placed in a cake tin. Carambola slices are lightly browned in butter and used for decoration.

It is then baked at 220°C for 10 minutes and then for another 15 minutes at 180°C until the cake is ready.

The cake is served hot or cold with whipped cream or ice cream.

Guava Strawberry Pie

2 cups ripe sliced guava
1 cup almonds
5 dried figs
5 strawberries
1 ripe banana
¼ cup honey

Almonds, figs and a bit of the honey are mixed together and filled into a pie plate. The guava, remaining honey, strawberries and banana are then mixed and poured into the pie shell and left in a refrigerator until set. Decorate with fruit slices and flaked almonds.

Guava Cocktail

½ cup Guava juice
½ cup pineapple juice
1 tablespoon lemon juice
1 tablespoon honey
a nip of rum
a nip of Cointreau

Mix all ingredients together well and fill into a high glass together with ice and decorate with orange slice.

Guava Desert

1½ cups guava pulp
2 avocados
3 mandarins
2 bananas
1 tablespoon brandy
3 tablespoons Cointreau
1 teaspoon Amaretto (Italian almond liqueur)
lemon juice and honey to taste
whipped cream and almond flakes for decoration

Avocados, mandarins and bananas are skinned and chopped into small pieces. The alcohol is poured over it and left to soak. The guava pulp is then mixed with honey and stirred in and filled into dessert dishes decorated with whipped cream and almond flakes.

Guava as Medicine

Using herbs to treat illnesses is as old as the existence of human beings. Even meat-consuming animals like cats and dogs cure themselves by eating grass.

Primitive medicine was built up on experience, and written down as on the clay boards of the Persian Gulf, which date back to around 4000BC. Other descriptions of medicinal plants in central Europe date back 3000 years.

The people from old Babylon already knew preparations of plants such as mustard seeds against toothache, which where documented around 2000BC. The priest and doctor Imhotep, the father of old Egyptian medicine, prescribed in 2500BC to the construction workers at the pyramids, daily rations of radish, onions and garlic as a protection against infectious diseases. At his time, approximately 250 medicinal plants like aniseed, fennel, coldsfoot, calamus, myrrh, linseeds, junipers and many others were used to treat diseases.

The first herb gardens with garlic, onions, fennel, saffron, thyme, mustard, caraways and dill emerged around 700BC.

The curative effects of plants and herbs observed over thousands of years, makes their application medically justifiable even if the efficacy is scientifically not yet proven.

There is an extensive treasure of undocumented knowledge on ancient traditional healing still practised by the natives, like the people of the Amazon or Aborigines of Australia, who could not write. Rain forest with its hundreds of thousands of different plants is an especially rich reservoir of valuable medicine. Only very little of it has been studied.

The guava is one of these plants, which drew attention only in recent times, despite guava being used successfully for many thousands of years for therapeutic purposes.

Guava has been used for many thousands of years as a sweet and fruity remedy by different Indians of middle and south America.

Particularly the fruit and the leaves have demonstrated a long history of a most curative effect.

The tea made from guava leaves has been valued throughout history against stomach-intestinal disorders, diarrhoea and inflammations.

Guava—A Healing Remedy Worldwide

Cuba: Cold, stomach and intestinal disorders.

Ghana and Central Africa: Toothache, wounds, intestinal cramps, diarrhoea, rheumatism, vertigo, nausea, kidney infections, colds, mouth inflammations, fevers, epilepsy, cholera, bronchitis, coughs and colds, insomnia and the leaves against worms.

Malaysia: Dermatitis, hysteria, epilepsy, diarrhoea, emmenagogue fevers.

Phillipines: Wounds, sores, astringent, childbirth. Fruit juice to strengthen the heart.

Trinidad: Diarrhoea, stomach and intestinal disorders (infusion)

Haiti: Stomach and intestinal disorders, antiseptic, astringent diarrhoea, piles, wounds, skin diseases, epilepsy

New Guinea: Against itching insect bites.

Tonga: Stomach-aches.

Tahiti: Skin tonic.

West Indian Islands: Epilepsy, coughs.

Brazil: Haemorrhoids, mouth inflammations, diarrhoea.

China: Diabetes.

Mexico: Stomach-aches, diarrhoea (Infusion from leaves and bark), ulcers and wounds, swellings.

Hawaii: Diarrhoea (chew the fresh young leaves)

Chile and Peru: Chewing the leaves for the strengthening of the gums.

Panama: Chew the leaves against toothache.

Samoa: The leaves as cough medicines and as an antidote against all kinds of poisonings

Asia: In some south Asian countries as well as in China a narcotic psidium drug is produced by feeding exclusively guava leaves to insects, particularly to grasshoppers. The excrement of the insects is collected, kneaded to small balls, dried and stored airtight. Some of these "pills" are dissolved in hot water and taken if required.

Science Discovered the Healing Power of Guava

Recent research into guava as medicine shows far greater effects than assumed.

A comprehensive study with Taiwanese guava clearly showed that guava juice can reduce the blood sugar level by up to 20%, taking 1gm of juice per kg body weight.

In Mexico, a country where treatment with guava have been traditional for thousands of years, a study proved that guava lowers the stool frequency and is therefore beneficial against mortality caused by diarrhoea. The study demonstrated clearly the benefits in the treatment of diarrhoea.

Considering that every year 5 million children are dying from diarrhoea at an age below one year, guava could be an affordable, safe and efficient treatment.

A study in Malaysia with rats demonstrated how artificially induced diarrhoea was cured within a few hours with guava leaf extract. It was found the extract is especially active in the small intestines, where a reduction of water secretion of 65% was measured (*Journal of Ethnopharmacology* 37 (1992) 151–157).

The prominent journal *Asia Pacific Journal of Pharmacology* (8 (1993) 83–87) published a research article using male albino mice which showed a morphine-like pain-blocking effect administrating guava leaves extract, injected under the skin. The mice treated with guava leaves displayed the comparable pain resistance as the mice pretreated with morphine at the "acid test" the "tail-clip test" and at the "hot panel".

This pain-killing effect is linked to the flavonoid "Quercetin" with its pain-killing properties, which is very similar to morphine.

Guava as a "painkiller" is increasingly more utilised by modern medicine in Malaysia.

Another study with mice at the University of Penang in Malaysia confirmed a clear analgesic, narcotic and relaxing effect. This study verified for the first time the effectiveness of guava leaves in the treatment of epilepsy, which natives in many countries have claimed for a long time.

These, as well as all the other studies, should teach us that the observations of natives over thousands of years are valuable knowledge, which should be investigated more for our benefits.

A study from Guatemala was able to confirm the antibacterial activity of the guava against pathological bacteria in the intestines, an effect known by the natives in Central America since ancient times as a treatment of intestine disorders.

An Indian study published in the *Journal of Human Hypertension* (7 (1993) 33–38) confirmed that the guava fruit has a decreasing effect in cases of high blood pressure and high blood fat readings. Over a period of 4 weeks, 2 groups with 73 patients each, who suffered from high blood pressure and high fat, received different diets. After 4 weeks it showed clearly, that the patients in the group who ate ½ to 1kg guava fruit daily, decreased their blood pressure by an average of 5%. Their fat readings also decreased by an average of 5–8%.

Another study from India published in the well-known journal *American Journal of Cardiology* (70 (1992) 1287–1291) reported similar results. Over a period of 12 weeks a diet high in fibre, and rich in guava fruit had a lowering effect on blood pressures in average of 9mm Hg. Simultaneously the cholesterol readings reduced by 9.9% and the triglycerid level by 7.7% while the so-called "good fats" (HDL) increased by over 8%.

A study by the University of Shizuoka in Japan, published in *Phytochemistry* 36 (1994) 1027–1029, the discovery of a substance in guava leaves, the so-called Gallocatechin. This substance has a particular antimutagene effect. That means, it is capable of repairing mutated DNA, damaged by poisons or radiation.

This ability to restore disturbed or changed gene structures will become in the future more and more important in regard to chemotherapy and treatment of cancer. The study clearly shows that the component Gallocatechin guava leaf tea is an active "bio-antimutagene" agent.

In *Food Chemical News* (31.7.95) a study from America was published, reporting the cancer-preventing effect of the guava fruit. According to the report, the guava fruit has on the one hand a cancer-preventing component, on the other hand cancer-promoting substances are blocked in their cell damaging action like nitrosamine (produced by frying and barbecuing). This anticarcinogene effect is linked to several substances in the guava fruit.

A study by a group of scientists at the Canadian University of Ottawa (*Record of Medical Research* 25 (1994) 11–15) was able to isolate from guava leaves the bioflavinoid "Quercetin" as well as five other important glycosides. They confirmed that the Quercetin and the Quercetin glycosides found in guava leaves are responsible for strong anti-spasm properties.

If it is administered to treat diarrhoea it can prevent the life endangering dehydration of the body.

Another study from Malaysia confirms the pain killing properties of guava leaves which are similar to morphine and linked also to the high content of Quercetin.

Extensive research by the University of Rome found that Quercetin is able to prevent breast cancer and to stop the growing of breast cancer cells. This happens by stimulating the body's own defence, the so-called Adriamycins.

A study published in *International Journal of Cancer* 54 (1993) confirms as well the ability of Quercetin to stop cancer cell growth especially in breast cancer.

A further important study about the effectiveness of Quercetins was published in the *Journal of Rheumatology* 24 (1997). There it is reported that Quercetin is in a position to block the so-called Tumor Necrose Factor a. This has far-reaching consequences in the therapy of rheumatoid arthritis, since the TNF is responsible is for the painful inflammation reactions.

All parts of plants from the root up to the tips of the leaves, including the blossoms and fruit, have a high medical value with wide spectrum effects.

All parts of the plant can be used—the flesh of the ripe fruit and the immature fruit, the skin of the immature fruit, the blossoms (as flower essences), the leaves, the seeds, the bark and even the roots.

Composition and Operation

Fruit: Water 76%, protein 1–5%, fat 0–2%, carbohydrates: 5–14%, calcium 0–0.1%, phosphorus 0–0.4%, irons 1mg/100gm, vitamin C 300–1000mg/100g

Besides the Indian gooseberry (Amla), no other fruit contains so much natural vitamin C as the guava. The fruit has its highest contents on vitamin C when fully ripe. The bark is very high in vitamin C as well. 100ml of the pure juice contain 70–170mg vitamin C, but is also rich in vitamin A and B as well as glycosides and enzymes.

Ripe guava has a pH of 3–4.

Guava is a slightly acid forming food, with a calcium (23mg/100g)-phosphorus (42mg/100g) ratio of 0.55 and is in this regard similar to soymilk, with a ratio of 0.51. Compared with avocado which is a very sour fruit with a ratio of 0.23 and cauliflower with a ratio of 0.44. Spinach is on the other hand and with a ratio of 3.00 and rhubarbs of 5.33 very alkaline forming (Aihara).

Guava has a very high content on lutein and zeaxanthin as well as lycopene. These are carotenes especially beneficial for eye diseases since they are regenerating the cells necessary to see. There is no other food known, which displays so high a content of these carotenes.

Leaves: Tannin (up to 10%), Seponin, Sitosterol, Maslen acid, Guaijavol acid, essential oils (mainly caryophyllen), chlorophyll, carotin, Quercetin glycoside, Amygdalin.

Effect: astringent, bactericidal, reassuring, pain blocking, narcotic, immune system supporting, anti-hypertensive, blood sugar and fat decreasing, disinfecting.

How to Make and Use Your Own Guava Medicine

Conservation of Guava

People in tropical countries never worry too much about conserving food since there are always fresh supplies available in the garden, from the bushes and trees or the local produce stored all year round. They just use the fruits in season. Banana, Papaya and Guava bear fruit all the year round. Conservation of fruits and leaves is however very important for those people who are not lucky enough to live in the tropics.

Preservation of fruit and leaves without destroying valuable components is especially important, if they are used for healing. Plant medicine must come only from biological cultures.

Juice: Guavas are first planted for the manufacture of the delightful, healthy juice.

Similarly like the fig, the ripe guava has only a very short shelf life. That is the reason why guava is seldom offered in green grocery shops. The purchase of guava juice or puree is therefore the best way for people living in non-tropical areas to enjoy guava which is especially appreciated by diabetics knowing about this beneficial side effect. Certainly, the leaves are not the best tasting like the fruit nectar. But the leaves have a higher medicinal value than the juice and are mixed with the juice as medicine against diabetes in Asia.

Drying: Young leaves are harvested and quickly dried in the shade. The drying temperature should not be over 45 degrees. Too low a temperature and too high a humidity should be avoided since mould could develop. Since the leaves dry faster than the stalks, the stalks are cut from the leaves and dried separately. It is recommended to cut or chop the stalk to ensure faster drying. The dried Guava are then rubbed or cut into small pieces and the leaf is used for tea. The tea should be stored in an airtight and if possible, glass container in a dark, cool place.

Water is the main ingredient of the leaves and fruit. To manufacture 1kg tea, one requires approximately 11 kg fresh leaves, or 13kg fresh fruit.

Applications of fresh leaves or fruit can be converted with these figures easily.

Careful Drying but Without Microwave: Drying with microwave is sometimes recommended. Certainly, the advantages are fastest drying, conservation of the colour, low temperatures the guarantee that no mould will develop.

Is cooking and herb drying with microwaves safe?

To say it in the shortest way possible, the answer is No. Reports warning of the dangers of Microwave ovens were published shortly after these speedy cookers were invented. Powerful industries have more money to invest in research which brings the scientific proof that microwave devices are safe. Are we not told that electricity is safe? The evidence that our modern helpers are making us ill is self-evident.

Since human beings first appeared on this earth they fed themselves with only fresh food, not manufactured, homogenised, microwaved and so on. This was living food with life energy in it. This life-force, energy, soul or what ever you may call it of food is destroyed by microwaving. OK, scientists find microwaving a perfect way of food preparation and energy saving on top of it. But are these scientists able to measure the life force? The answer is easy "there is no life force", say scientists.

Maybe you would like to do your own research.

Take 2 flowerpots, fill them both with potting mix from one batch and put seeds in it from the same batch and put the seeds from the same packet in them. Next, heat one pot in the microwave oven to say 80°C and the other pot in a conventional heater to exactly the same temperature. Water both pots with the same care for the next few weeks. You will be able to measure the life force by a simple method: the pot heated with a conventional heater will produce nice plants, the pot heated with the microwave oven has only stinking rotten seeds in it. Even if we cannot find the life force, we can prove that it is destroyed with the modern microwaves which converts healthy food into dead food. Think about it!

The fruit is washed, cut open in quarters. The fruit should be dried as quickly as possible in the shade or in a stove, at a temperature of maximum 45°C. Heating panels, as used for beer brewing, are ideal as well as for drying of the leaves and seed.

After the fruit have dried well, they are stored immediately in airtight containers in a cool place. In Asia, particularly China, a mixture of dried fruit and leaves are taken as an effective, pleasant tasting blend against diabetes.

Dried fruit as well as leaves are chewed against inflammations in the mouth and against toothaches.

Seeds can be dried separately from the fruit flesh. Like the leaves, they are also dried in the shade or at low temperature in the oven and stored airtight in a cool place. They may later be used for sowing. In Malaysia, the seeds are chewed against constipation. However, caution should be taken since in other countries people are told that they should not eat guavas when suffering from constipation but there is no mention of chewed guava seeds.

Wine: Some people make very pleasant tasting guava wine from the ripe fruit. Wine from strawberry guava tastes more heartily and spicier than the wine from ordinary guava.

Beer from guava has a good taste. It is similar to wheat beer. If anyone has problems with the froth of wheat beer, they should not have guava beer, since this has more foam.

The Best Preservation: Lactic Acid Fermentation

The term lactic acid fermentation does not sound very appetising. The products associated with this term however are not only well known but also very popular. What would we do without wine, beer and cheese on our menu? The lactic acid fermentation process is an important part in preservation. One of the best examples of this fermentation process is sauerkraut. The famous sea captain, Captain Cook, took sauerkraut with him on his expedition as this was the only way to preserve vitamins in those times. Without the important vitamin C (approximately 20mg per 100gm of sauerkraut) the men on those ships would have contracted scurvy. Not only vitamin C is conserved with lactic acid fermentation but also the vitamins A, B1, B2, B6, B12, D, E, K and even more are produced during the lactic acid fermentation process. Of course sauerkraut then is not necessarily the same as sauerkraut of today. Today salt is mostly used in sauerkraut. In the early days, people used less salt and therefore more herbs and spices, such as juniper berry, mustard seed and thyme. To avoid calcium deficiency, it was common to add eggshell flour to the sauerkraut.

Sauerkraut is a very effective herb and it is not only a food mainly eaten by the Germans. Sauerkraut means sour-herb. For treatments, sauerkraut should not be cooked as it is with sausages and pork roast in Germany. Temperature over 45°C destroys the ferments. It is similar to the way it is with milk. Cooked, pasturised, homogenised milk is harder to digest than raw milk. Sour milk or even better Kefir fermented milk is easy to digest since fermentation pre-digests it.

Sauerkraut increases the blood circulation of the intestines and is one of the best remedies for chronic constipation. Sauerkraut should be in every slimming diet to avoid negative side effects.

Guava Sauer-Herb Fermentation

Most herbs are suitable for the lactic acid fermentation process. However some ferment easier than others. You can mix herbs together which you harvest on the same day such as Dandelion, Lady's Bedstraw, Balm, knotgrass, Raspberry leaves, Peppermint, ribwort Plantain and other herbs which grow around your area or you may want to get them out of your garden. Only mix together herbs that are beneficial. You may add small quantities of dill seeds, mustard seeds or bay leaves. Wormwood for a better taste, century and other very bitter herbs should not be added, they could make the total mixture very bitter.

For lactic acid fermentation everything has to be absolutely clean. The herbs are washed, chopped like parsley and crushed with a rolling pin and put in the fermenting container. Press the herbs in the container as hard as you can. This is very important. I remember as a child that we had to tread the cabbage in the 50-litre containers with our bare feet—washed before of course. Add clean water with salt (avoid the use of free flowing salt) so that the herbs are submerged. The amount of salt depends on the weight of herbs you have in the container and should be 1% or 1gm or 10gm per kilo. Commercial sauerkraut has 3% salt which you could use for your first try as well. With some experience you may go as low as 0.3%. Two little boards with holes (for the fingers to get it out again) are placed on top of the herbs. A rock (sterilised in boiling water before use) is placed on top of the two little boards to weigh them down. An airtight lid covers the pot. For the first 8–10 days a temperature of 20–25°C is recommended. After this first part of fermentation the pot is placed in a cool place. After 6 weeks you may start using the herbs but it is better to wait until 8 weeks.

Fermentation with the Kombucha Culture
For beginner this is the easier way of lactic acid fermentation. You may use different herbal teas and ferment this to your taste or needs. You may use dried herbs or fresh herbs as if you were making herbal tea for immediate consumption. Add sugar and Kombucha tea culture and ferment as you normally brew your Kombucha.

Lactic acid fermented food is pro-biotic which means live promoting.

For further reading about lactic acid fermented food it is recommended to read the following books: *Kombucha The miracle Fungus, Kombucha Teaology, Kefir for pleasure and well-being and Herbal Teology*.

Presumably you will wonder what all that has to do with guava. Very simple, from guava leaves and fruits one can manufacture lactic acid fermented guavas. In this way the food keeps its pro-biotic power. This makes chemical preservatives, high heat or better still over heating, irradiation, etc. unnecessary. Fresh, alive, lactic acid fermented foods like sauerkraut, or in this case sour guava, support the digestion. In the lactic acid fermentation process not only vitamins are produced, but also friendly bacteria, which we need in our digestive tract. With antibiotics the pathogenic or ill-provoking bacteria are destroyed but also the good or friendly bacteria, the probiotics, which are necessary for digestion and for the immune system to fight disease. A person with a disturbed intestinal flora cannot be healthy. If it is unavoidable to take antibiotics, to save life, one should take pro-biotic foods like yoghurt, buttermilk, Kefir, Kombucha after treatment.

The efficacy of plant medicine depends considerably on their freshness. Guava has only a very short shelf life and fresh leaves are available only in tropical countries. But even there it is very difficult for people living in cities to obtain fresh leaves from organic production.

Guava-Papaya-Concentrate

In many countries, east and west alike, Australian Guava-Papaya-Concentrate is available. It is a successful development of Josè Perko (The Kombucha House Queensland, Australia). Mr. Perko combined the two outstanding medicinal plants, Guava and Papaya, and refined and enhanced their healing properties through a lactic acid fermentation process developed over years. With this process, the healing properties are conserved for long-term storage. Lactic acid fermented food increases these properties so that they are more easily absorbed into the body.

A Particularly Good Combination: Guava-Papaya-Concentrate

Papaya is the best fruit for good digestion. Papaya is rich in digestive enzymes. Papaya can help to balance diet sins. After a meal that is hard to digest it is recommended you have papaya as a dessert or a cup of Papaya tea to help the digestion (or indigestion) that one feels long after a heavy meal. Taken over a long period of time Papaya can also help to correct years of dietary mistakes. Mucous in the intestines which negatively influence our digestion can be reduced and even intestinal parasites digested. For indigestion the Papaya should be consumed together with the seeds. Many specialists consider papain as the strongest protein digesting enzyme. Papain, the super enzyme, can digest 35 times its own weight in meat. Papain is active in the digestive system in sour, alkaline or neutral surroundings. For people who do not produce enough stomach acid, their own produced protein-digesting enzyme pepsin is not active enough. The strong protein-digesting enzyme papain can help here.

Mucous built up in the intestine can be the cause of low energy, poor digestion and other illnesses. Partly digested protein stays in the intestinal walls and hinders proper digestion. Papain can digest the different proteins so that they do not block digestion and reduce, over a longer period of time, the existing build up. Papain can therefore be seen as an excellent body cleansing agent, breaking down hard-to-digest protein and setting free amino acid Alanine to strengthen the cell walls for example.

Inefficient protein digestion may also be responsible for arthritis, constipation, diabetes, high blood pressure and so on. Being healthy and staying healthy depends initially on the strength of our immune system. Papain sets amino acids free, detoxifies the body and in this way strengthens the body's own immune system and can be seen as a first class healer.

In the concentrate the Papaya complements effects offered by guava. One has astonishing successes particularly with pancreas disorders like diabetes, with diarrhoea, gastritis, digestive troubles, heartburn, constipation, swellings and inflammations, throat complaints, rheumatism, pain, stress and toothaches.

For further reading the book *Papaya The Medicine Tree* by Harald Tietze is recommended.

Guava Preparations

Go by your own feeling and needs. For daily use an infusion of the leaves or dried fruit is most common.

Decoction of Guava—Boil up 1–2 handfuls of chopped leaves in water for 5 minutes. Cool and use as a skin wash and lotion. Beneficial to treat impetigo, itching skin, rashes, scabies, skin sores, pimples, psoriasis, superficial cuts and wounds.

Guava Tea from Leaves (cut or pulverised)

Guava-Tea is prepared like other herb tea. Guava Tea prices vary tremendously. Sometimes cheap teas are offered from strawberry guava. Medicinal effects of this tea are not known. Good teas from young leaves and biological produce are of course expensive, but better.

Guava leave tea tastes very nice, if one considers that it is a medicinal tea. For better taste the tea from ripe fruit is the best. However, this tea has not the medicinal value that the leaves have.

To cure diseases with tea, the tea itself, the tea leaves should be taken so that one does not throw away the most valuable part. Guava leaves are very leathery and tough, and therefore it is not easy to consume the tea leaves. Leaf powder is easier to use as salad dressing. In this way other beneficial components are utilised by the body.

Beside the leaf tea there are also mixtures from leaves and fruit, which are taken in as a remedy against diabetes.

Guava Leaves Powder is manufactured in Australia from biologically grown young guavas. One uses the powder for tea, whereby one drinks or eats the powder with the tea or with the salad and does not throw valuable leaves away. Guava powder is also used for body and beauty care.

Guava Fruit Powder
Use fresh fruit, discard the seeds and sun-dry the fruit then grind to a powder.

Can be used for impetigo, prickly heat rash, head sores, boils and wounds.

Why do Bees Love Guava Leaves?

Guava leaves when dried, are very hard. I (Harald) drink the leaves with my herbal teas, since in my opinion the most valuable elements of the tea are in the leaves and should not be thrown away.

My friend Jose mills guava tea leaves extremely fine, so that it is easier to swallow the tea without hurting the mucous membranes. Jose observed something unusual. He worked over decades with herbs and is an experienced beekeeper as well.

Something unusual happens when he mills guava leaves. 100–150 bees come from around the area to the finely woven bag which catches the tea. Only very fine guava dust is able to go through the fabric. The bees quickly carry this fine guava dust away.

I personally produced in my medicinal nursery over many years 56 different medicinal herbal teas, and used the same method to mill the tea. My neighbour is also a beekeeper and the bees always came to the flowers of my plants, but never to carry away dust from the bags. Guava can be a strange exception and we cannot explain why the bees are carrying the dust and not the nectar from the flowers which were in abundance around at the time of milling. Something in the fine guava dust must have attracted the bees strongly.

Guava Lotion
Use 500gm of fresh guava, cover with water and simmer until liquid thickens. Alternatively use 50gm of dried fruit with ½ litre water.

Can be used to treat acne, boils, eczema, impetigo, head sores, pimples, prickly heat rash and puritis. Apply lotion to affected areas 2–3 times a day.

Guava Skin Extract (in water)
Guava is a potent medicinal plant. The skin of the ripe fruit is considered similar to the leaves in having the highest healing power. Instead of throwing the skin away, as is usually, it is put into a glass jar and filled with enough water to cover the skins well. The glass container is then covered with a cloth (cheesecloth or a fine fabric) and the fabric is sealed with a rubber ring on top of the glass. This enables the brew to breathe and prevent insects from getting into the jar. The jar is then placed in natural light (sunlight) for 24 hours. There is still enough sunlight on a cloudy day. At night the moonlight should

reach the glass—moonlight is nothing else but reflected sunlight.

After 24 hours the beverage is ready and it is taken among other things to quench the thirst of the diabetics.

Guava Oil
Everyone can produce his/her own oil. Normally the skin or the leaf is used, cut into small pieces and placed in a pot (not aluminium). Using dried leaf tea, which is ground very fine, one must consider that dried leaves weigh only 10% as the same amount of fresh leaves. Olive oil is then added so that all pieces are well covered. The oil is simmered for approximately 5 minutes. The oil with the leaves or the skin is stored for 2 days before it is pressed out. To press out the oil one can squeeze out the plant parts in a towel. The squeezed plant parts as well as the oil is used mainly externally for massages against pain and should be part of every massage oil mixture.

Guava Leaves and Fruit Skin Compresses
Mainly the leaves and the skin of the fruit are used. The leaves or skin are poulticed, the same as you do with cabbage leaves, and placed on the affected areas. Compresses are applied hot or cold depending on the illness.

Pickled Guava in Salt
The fruit (with the skin) is cut into thin slices or grated and placed into a glass jar. Salt water (3% or 30gm salt

per litre of water) is then added until the guava is well covered. The jars are then stored in a cool place for maturing.

Pickled Guava in Vinegar

The fruit (with the skin) is cut into thin slices. A glass jar is two-thirds filled with the Guava. Vinegar is then poured over until it is well covered. Guava vinegar can be stored for a very long time.

Guava Vinegar

The vinegar of the pickled papaya, as above, has to mature for a minimum of six weeks and is then strained. One can produce one's own vinegar by using the Kombucha brewing method. Instead of using black or green tea as is usual with Kombucha brewing, guava tea is used instead. Mixing both teas together works very well. The skins of the guava can be used for the vinegar production as well.

Instead of fermenting, as is usual with Kombucha for only 1–2 weeks, this vinegar needs to ferment for at least 6 weeks to become vinegar.

This Kombucha guava vinegar can be used like usual vinegar to maintain health or for the treatment of illnesses.

Guava-Kombucha-Culture Compress against Pains

The fungus, as it is called, is a lichen and grows on the surface of the Kombucha brew.

Brewing Kombucha with different medicinal herbs produces different structures of Kombucha cultures. A brew with guava tea produces the toughest culture. Such a dried culture is like leather. In comparison the culture from a papaya brew is very soft and often falls apart when removing from a large container.

A fresh guava culture is an excellent treatment against pain like it is with arthritis or rheumatism.

Some people achieved incredible successes with this treatment, when pain made it necessary to go on crutches. With only one, or in some cases two treatments with Kombucha culture compresses, these people were able to live a bearable life. The entire fluid of the culture is absorbed in the skin over several hours. A culture, 10mm thick, is as thin as paper the next morning.

Caution: This treatment could have bad side effects. The culture, and with it the fluid, has a pH of about 3 and is very sour. Some people, who tried many other treatments unsuccessfully had spontaneous successes with the Kombucha culture compress, but left it on the skin too long. The consequence was that an itching rash developed at the previously sore place. All people who reported similar effects complained about the unpleasant itching, which stops after a few hours but also can last up to two days. Despite this undesirable side effect, some commented that they were happy to swap intolerable pain for itchiness.

However, this undesirable complaint can be excluded, if one examines the skin under the culture every 20 minutes. After 20 minutes some people react with red skin and the treatment should be discontinued. Such a fast reaction is rare, but a woman had this experience in an effort to look very attractive for a particular evening. She works in a clinic and had learnt from the patients about the application for younger looking blooming skin. She blended a culture and used it on her face. After 20 minutes she looked not blooming but glowing, and had to cover the error with makeup!

An 80-year-old woman who had a problem with her foot left a Kombucha culture compress on the foot for one whole night. Next morning the complaint had almost completely disappeared. The same treatment was repeated the next night with better success for the problem but with itching side effect. Most probably she should have had the treatment only for a few hours more and not for the whole night.

The culture should not be placed in the hair!

The culture is very popular as a facemask. For this purpose it is made to a cream in a blender. Neither the cream nor the whole fungus may be used in hairy places, since it immediately sticks to the hair and cannot be removed. No shampoo helps to remove the culture particles. Some women, who wanted to be especially beautiful, used the culture in their hair and ended up with an unwanted haircut or unintentionally thinned eyebrows.

However, some women use the culture to remove undesirable hair on the legs or lips.

If someone wants to use the culture creams where there is hair, some drops of olive oil prevent the culture from attaching. The woman from America who told me about this preventive treatment did not reveal to me the exact ratio used. She used blended culture especially for the hair care for her favourite dog.

Bathing in Guava Vinegar
Two cups of guava vinegar is added to a full bath or ¼ cup to a shallow bath.

If the concentrate is used, this must be diluted accordingly.

Bathing in Guava vinegar is analgesic and calming. A mixture with St. John's Wort (tea or vinegar) enhances the effect.

Compresses with Guava Vinegar
The effectiveness of remedies using an external application is mostly underestimated.

Compresses work through the skin but without affecting the digestive system.

A mixture is made of ¼ litre of guava vinegar and ¾ litre of water. A cotton towel is soaked in the diluted vinegar, lightly wrung out and placed on the problem area. A plastic wrap-like Glad Wrap is then placed on top of the compress to avoid the vinegar disappearing in the wrong direction. A larger dry towel is then laid over the compress to avoid cooling.

Guava Tincture
The skin or young leaves are used to produce a guava tincture. Using the skin, the fruit flesh is removed. The skin or leaves are then placed in the jar. If you use the tincture afterwards as mother tincture for producing homeopathic medicine—new jars should be used, since cucumber or sauerkraut jars are not suitable. Alcohol, such as Vodka, is poured over, or if available, pure alcohol diluted down to 40% so that the leaves or skin are well covered. The glass is then shaken every day over a period of 4–6 weeks. After that time, the tincture is then sieved but one can leave the skin or leaves in the tincture and use the tincture whenever needed. The tincture has a long shelf life over many years and can be taken when needed. To produce homeopathic guava medicine different plant parts may be used to produce the mother tincture as above. The first preference is to use the young leaves.

Fresh green guavas and leaves taste good. The advantage of homeopathic guava is that it has a long shelf life and no sign of bitterness due to dilution.

Homeopathic Guava

One can use as mother tinctures for the above, guava tincture.

The principle of homeopathic medicine is only the information (homeopathic frequency) of the medicine, the information of the herb instead of the herb itself. The homeopathic tincture is placed under the tongue and is not swallowed like beer but kept as long as possible in the mouth and swallowed naturally after a while.

How homeopathic medicine works is not fully understood but the results cannot be ignored.

The mechanism of homeopathic medicine may be explained with some recent research in Japan in regard to urine therapy. Tests have shown that urine applied directly into the stomach through a tube had no effect in cancer treatment but oral application showed good results. The fact that cancer occurs in the bladder, urinary tract and kidneys proves that the presence of urine inside the body does not have any direct effect on carcinogenic cells. But when the same urine is taken orally and passes through the throat, a decrease in carcinogenic cell growth or the disappearance of cancer has been observed in some cancer patients.

Even if urine is not ingested but only gargled, the effects were found to be the same as when it was ingested.

Because of the above findings, it can be assumed that sensor cells which can perceive extremely minute changes in the body, could control them if stimulated by the right information from urine. Such cells are found in the oral cavity and throat, said Dr Ryoichi Nakao, Chairman of the M.C.L Institute of Japan in his speech at the first world conference on urine therapy in Goa, India 1996.

Making homeopathic medicine is easy but time-consuming and one has to follow exact procedures.

How to Make Homeopathic Guava Medicine

Homeopathic dilutions are calculated in D1, D6, D30 or anything in between. It means that one drop in ten drops in D1 and one drop in a million drops in D6 for example. D6 means dilution 6 times. D6 is sometimes called 6x which is the same. Do not think it is very difficult to get this dilution. You do not have to count 1,000,000 drops of water and add just 1 drop of guava tincture to it to get it right. There is a simple system to it. If you want to make homeopathic medicine it is advisable to buy, at the pharmacist or chemist, six small test tubes (you may also use other little glass containers like little bottles) and a medicine dropper.

a. Put all the six test tubes in some kind of a stand, maybe a little pot or a big mug, and put 9 drops of neutral water in every test tube, do not use tap water as it contains fluoride or chlorine, it is better to buy pure water.
b. The next step is to use one drop from the guava tincture and add it to the water in the first test tube. Clean the dropper, as it needs to be completely clean before you use it again and again.

c. Now take the test tube in your hand, with your thumb covering the opening, and shake the bottle 50 times. This is very important. What you have now is D1.
d. Now take one drop from your D1 and put it in the second test tube; do exactly the same procedure again, clean the dropper, shake 50 times and then you have homeopathic urine D2.
e. Next take one drop from this homeopathic urine D2 and put it in the third test tube. Do the same thing until you have repeated the whole procedure with your six bottles and now you have one drop of urine in 1,000,000 drops of water which is dilution 6 or D6 or 6x homeopathic guava.

The above explains the principle on how to make homeopathic dilutions. Certainly one can make larger quantities by using drops instead of millilitres, for example 90ml water to which 10ml tincture is added.

You can make your own homeopathic medicine from other herbs as well using one drop of mother tincture. Please make absolutely sure that you use only the best quality ingredients for your tincture. The product you produce yourself is then the best, grown in your area, with best quality ingredients and made with love and care.

To store homeopathic medicine over a longer period of time it is advisable to use pure alcohol, preferably in the last test tube. If you cannot get pure alcohol at your chemist you may also use vodka, or Slivovics or other fruit alcohol.

For the beginner maybe it sounds a little bit difficult, but when you have done it a few times you will find out that it is a very simple procedure. If you are interested in finding out more about homeopathic medicine please contact Harald W. Tietze Publishing and ask for the book list. There are some very good books about homeopathy for the beginner and the therapist available like *Beginners Guide to Homeopathy* (518 pages) by T.S. Iyer and *Practice of Homeopathy at Home* (601 pages) by Dr B.B. Jadhav.

Guava Flower Essence

Flower essences have been used for rituals and healing by natives down through the ages and have just been rediscovered in the last decades. The best known of these are the 38 Bach Flower Essences named after the homeopath Dr Edward Bach (1886-1936) who lived in Mount Vernon in England. Flower essences work on the psychological and intellectual levels as a preventative measure or to treat illness in a holistic approach.

Flower essences work in a similar manner to homeopathic medicine with the frequency or vibration of the plant and rather than through any so-called active ingredients. Usually, natural or chemical medicine is only taken to treat illness, but flower essences are suitable to maintain health and to work in a gentle way for the body and mind, to avoid manifestation of disorders. When needed, a number of drops are placed under the tongue several times daily according to directions or needs. As with homeopathic medicine, flower essences are not swallowed, but kept, for best results, as long as possible in the mouth under the tongue.

The Stepanovs Method

In the normal manner of producing flower essences, flowers are picked, placed in a bowl of water and left for 3 hours in the sun. The flowers are then removed and the water is then mixed with Cognac to make the mother tincture.

Juta Stepanovs has worked with plants for a number of years and through her connection with them has developed the concept of not destroying or disturbing the flowers in their natural environment whilst still maintaining the living vibrational energy in the flower essences. She was inspired by the method used by Aborigines to produce flower essences. They did not cut the flower but simply poured water continuously over them and collected it in a bowl. This procedure was repeated a number of times using the same water.

The second concern of Juta Stepanovs with the common way of producing flower essences was the quality of the water used. Nobody could answer her questions clearly on the best water to produce the essences? Is it pure dead water H_2O, rainwater, bore water or sterile tap water with all the chemicals added today? Her aim was to make essences with living water.

In the Stepanovs method, the flowers are not cut and placed into water, but the living water is collected from the flower itself, or from other parts of the plant. This method is extremely time consuming, since some flowers, especially from plants growing in a dry environment, yield only a few ml per day, however, the plants love this method and this is clearly visible after the collecting containers are removed. This extract of the plant is called the Alpha-essence.

Advantages of the Stepanovs Method

- The flower of the plant is not cut off and can complete its natural cycle after harvesting of the essence.
- The vibrational frequencies of the flowers or plant parts are living and not in the first stages of death.
- Alpha-essence, collected with the Stepanovs method, is 100% plant extract.
- With the Stepanovs method the specific, living essence, the pure Alpha-essence is extracted.

For the production of guava flower essences only flowers from wild guavas are used. Flowers from commercial plantations and from fruit without seeds are not suitable for flower essences. Trees from plantations, even when grown biologically, are supported by weed control, cutting and watering in drying times. The wild tree on the other hand grows only where the location and the soil is suitable, where it can unfold in space, for nutrients and water in the competition with other plants. Only such plants who fight independently but develop well are the right basis can be for the production of essences.

Guava suits well to produce essence with the Stepanovs method.

Application of the Guava Flower Essence

Fruit with many seeds are always a sign of rich energy, which is offered in great numbers by the guava. The guava is therefore one of the richest plants for cosmic energy, and vigour.

The guava essence is used mainly for exhaustion through stress, nervousness, excitement and especially fear.

For further reading the book *Australian Bush Flower Essences—The Steanovs Method* is recommended. The book tells in an easy way on how to produce and use flower essences with the Stepanovs method.

Applications of Guava of A-Z

Disease is a disturbed internal balance. The cause of these disturbances is in most cases daily burdens, which the bodies own resistance power cannot handle anymore.

Some of these causes are:

1. Social e.g. Stress, overstrain and frustration at the job, with neighbours or the wife / husband, selfishness, intolerance, inflexibility
2. Psychological e.g. unprocessed conflicts and compunctions, self-hate, defect of self-love and self-confidence
3. Biological e.g. inefficient immunity due to wrong nourishment, lack of hardening, lack of exercise
4. Environmental e.g. environmental poisonings, air pollution, food and drug (social and medicinal) poisons.

Nevertheless diseases are, if one considers them holistic, also somehow positively purifying.

Diseases are engine on the way to a fulfilled life.

Until today, disease has been seen as the worst evil of this world. Science is researching and developing successfully new ways to fight and eliminates diseases. A fight however, which appears to never end, since for every conquered disease apparently another one emerges.

Like everything in the world, disease has two sides: A suffering one and an enriching one for further personal development.

Under this view, the horror part of disease disappears so that body and mind can concentrate on the cause of the unbalance for a long insightful path of individual development.

A person who acknowledges that disease is no coincidence, but a logical consequence of thinking and behaviour pattern, can see disease as a gift with the possibility to learn, understand and correct this wrong thinking and behaviour pattern. Disease is the signal and motivation factor our soul uses to show us mistakes and prevent in the long-term bigger damage.

It is very important to see disease under a holistic aspect since the best remedy—guava included—can only unfold their full healing power, if through a natural lifestyle all ill provoking elements are consequently eliminated.

The following are indications where guava was used with success over long period of time. Please note that the dosages mentioned are only guidelines. Please note that guava fruits and leaves may have different qualities depending on the origin of the product. We are all individuals and react differently. As with all other remedies one should trust ones own feelings when learning from other people's observations and experiences.

Acne
Three times daily Guava tea, additional Guava lotion applications. Inflammations are washed repeatedly with guava leaf infusion.

Other support: change of diet, Symbiotic Colon therapy, homeopathic Sulphur D6 and Silicea D12, washings with sea sand and almond meal, Hamamelis—or Arnica tincture.

Allergies-General

The best remedy against allergies is certainly the allergy causing substance itself in homeopathic dilution.

Beside that, Urintherapy is in many cases the only answer. There are several methods using urine therapy. Against allergies, homeopathic urine and the drop under the tongue method has proven in many cases to be the best remedy. This remedy is not only effective but also free and without negative side effects. For further reading on this unique therapy see the book by Harald Tietze, Urine the Holy Water. Guava can give support only through the beneficial effects on the intestines. Guava fruit, powders and tea work here stabilising the metabolic processes particularly in the intestines.

Other support: change of diet, Symbiotic Colon therapy and decontamination, Autohomological blood therapy, bee pollen, acupuncture.

Artheriosklerosis

Guava juice, Guava Skin Extract

Other support: Ginkgo, garlic, mistletoe and Soy-lecitin, bloodletting, change diet, Kneipp therapy, therapeutic exercise, Wiedemann's serum therapy, Ozone therapy.

Arthrose/Rheumatism

Guava-Kombucha-Concentrate, compresses with cooled down infusion (not hot), massages with guava lotion, when needed 3 cups of guava tea per day, guava leave compresses. See also under pain.

Other support: Stinging nettle high dosage, arnica, willow bark extract, harpagophytum procumbens.

Homeopathic: Pulsatilla, Bryonie.

Massages with St. John's Wort oil and tea tree oil, acupuncture, gymnastics, Kneipp therapy, Elektro therapie, Wiedemann's serum therapy.

Asthma

The ripe flesh with the seeds are eaten, "weak" guava tea sweetened with honey is taken three times daily. Guava leaf infusion for inhalation, followed compresses at the chest with this infusion.

Other support: Teas and Inhalation of coldsfoot, plantain, thyme, efeu, knotgrass (Knotweed), autohomological blood therapy, urine therapy, acupuncture.

Athlete's Foot

Footbaths with concentrated guava tea.

Other support: Symbiotic Colon therapy, juniper berry oil, Urine therapy, massages with tea tree oil.

Blood Cleansing

0.5–1kg Guava flesh, Guava vinegar is added to the bath water, 3 cups guava tea per day.

Other support: stinging nettle, artichoke, juice from fresh dandelion, raw food diet, water therapy with 3–4 litre per day.

Blood Pressure, too high
0.5 to a maximum of 1kg Guava flesh per day, 3x daily ¼ litre tea (doesn't have to be strong).
Other support: mistletoe, garlic, hawthorn, arnica, Blood letting, relaxation therapy, acupuncture.

Bleeding, stopping of
Compresses with young fresh guava leaves, washings with guava infusions

Bronchitis Warmed up juice of the ripe Guava, against frequent coughing fits drink tea regularly, see asthma.

Cancer-Guava and Treatment of Cancer
Cancer is caused by a multitude of triggering components:

Hereditary factor, viruses, environmental toxins, frequencies, magnetic fields, wrong diet, mutations, mechanical influences, psychogenic elements; influences at work, social, and climatic; earth energy lines, Karma and many other factors can lead to it, so that cancer cells multiply freely.

It must be the main goal of every holistic therapy to uncover the causes of the illness and consequently eliminate them. This makes it necessary in many cases that major changes have to be done to achieve an "optimal" natural lifestyle. Sufficient sleep, healthy nourishment, sufficient exercise, time for relaxation and meditation are only some of the elements which give the will the power to regain health.

If this will is strong, guava can be a valuable part of the treatment together with the other supplementary treatments to help the patient on his way to health and well-being. Two fruit should be eaten three times daily. An additional 2 or 3 cups of guava tea should be taken per day. Guava-Papaya-Kombucha concentrate (manufactured by the Kombucha House Australia) should be taken in addition regularly. Guava is, like Papaya, the perfect diet to support the body in its own fight against cancer. Already many people have found help with this special concentrate.

In addition other effective treatments should be utilised to raise the body's own self-healing power optimally.

1. Ozone-oxygen therapy with additional vitamin C (12–18 sessions/2x per year).
2. Oxygen-therapy by Ardenne (12–18 sessions/4–5x per year).
3. Hämatogene Oxidationstherapy (12 sessions/1x per year).
4. Ozone-autohomological blood therapy under addition of Echinacin.

5. Immune system stimulation through herbal preparations: Thuja, Eleutherococcus, Baptistaextract, Echinacea, Ginseng, Papaya among others (12–18 injections and oral).
6. *Organlysat-therapy*:
   a. *Thymusspezialkur* (15–18 sessions/2x per year) e.g. *Thymoject* of *biosyn*.
   b. Regimen with liver-spleen extracts (parallel to Chemotherapy) e.g. factor AF

Antroposophic Medicine
Interleukinmodulation through *Mistellektine* (7 injections, then 2-week break), for example, *Eurixor (biosyn)* or *Iscador*.

With Mistletoe therapy by Iscador one uses the entire plant *Viscum album*, however matching to the kind of cancer (according to the antroposophic doctrine) the mistletoe of different host plants like the following are used:

- Cancerous growths in the digestive system, the urinary tract and the extremities: mistletoe from the Apple tree for women and mistletoe from the oak tree for men.
- Cancerous growths of the nose area, throat and the skin: mistletoe from the Pine tree.

- Cancerous growths of the bronchi: mistletoe from the oak tree for men and for women mistletoe from the Pine and Elm.

7. Immune-therapy through trace elements particularly *Selen* (especially *Selenase*), zinc, coppers and Lithium
8. Substitutions-therapy with enzymes and vitamins, especially C and E.
9. Micro-biological therapy, Symbiotic Colon therapy.
10. Homeopathic therapies.
11. Food supplements like Papaja, Spirulina, Kombucha among others.
12. In special cases acupuncture and treatments of traditional Chinese medicine.

All these methods do not have to be applied alternatively. They all suit excellently as additional treatments (in addition to "chemotherapy and radiation").

Cramps
Applications of guava tincture at the affected area especially at night with cramps in the leg.

Other support: compresses with lemon balm, massages with tea tree oil. Homeopathic *nux vomica*

Dizziness
4–5 cups weak guava tea is taken per day. Guava D12, Guava Flower Essence.

Other support: Symbiotic Colon therapy, Gingko, Cactus, Hawthorn.

Homeopathic: *nux vomica*,

Exhaustion
Fresh Guava fruit and juices mixed with much water.

Additional support: Magnesium and vitamin E, Siberia Ginseng, Spirulina, Kombucha, Kneipp treatments

Disinfection
A strong tea is cooked from the young shoots (with leaves), which is used as a vaginal douche after birth. In the Philippines it is custom to use an odd number of leaves, such as 11 or 13. Even numbers bring no success, or misfortune. For small operations, like circumcision, this tea is utilised as well.

Depressions, Fears
Guava flower essences, 3 cups guava tea a day

Other support: St. John's Wort, lemon balm, figs, valerian, hops, Kava Kava, acupuncture, relaxation therapy.

Diabetes
Guava diet with 0.5–1kg flesh per day, 3 cups Guava leaf tea is taken (the tea with the leaves!) using 1 teaspoon pulverised tea per cup. Guava skin extract is a good thirst quencher and decreases additionally the blood sugar level and blood pressure.

Other support: diet adjustments, Symbiotic Colon therapy, therapeutic exercise, Indian Psyllium, water drink regimen 3–4 litre per day.

Diverticulitis
Caution: The seeds should not be eaten.

Long-term Guava diet with fruit and juices.

Other support: long-term papaya diet, Indian Psyllium, alder bark, senna, linseeds, aloe, Symbiotic Colon therapy, therapeutic exercise.

Diarrhoea
A handful of fresh guava leaves are heated up in ½ litre of water just to the boiling point than left for 5 minutes to settle. Several cups are taking a when needed. Guava tea power may be used for as well.

Other support: Oak bark, silverweed, agrimony, microbial therapy, Symbiotic Colon therapy.

Eczema
A helpful treatment by soaking into a bath to which you add ½ cup guava vinegar, ½ cup fine oatmeal, essential oils of juniper 2 drops, lavender 2 drops and geranium 2 drops.

Eczema Lotion
Guava oil 40ml, guava vinegar 10ml, essential oils bergamot 10 drops, lavender 8 drops, melissa 4 drops,

Chamomile 3 drops. Shake well before use and apply to affected areas twice a day.

Epilepsy
Massages along the spine with guava tincture, drinking of highly concentrated Tea made from guava tea powder (including the powder), guava tincture is added to the bathwater.

Other support: relaxation therapy, psychotherapy (Systemic family therapy by Hellinger)

Fevers
Guava diet, guava tea, guava tincture is added to the bath water, compresses at chest and lower legs with cold guava tea and vinegar.

Flatulence
Seeds are chewed well and swallowed, guava tea, Guava Skin Extract, guava leaf infusion for abdominal compresses, stomach massages with guava oil.

Other support: Indian Psyllium, boldo leaves, dill seeds, caraway, mint, abdominal massages with bergamot oil, warm compresses with camomile, change of diet, therapeutic exercise, Symbiotic Colon therapy.

Gout
Guava leaf tea, whole fruit, cold guava tea compresses. See also Rheumatism and Pain.

Hair Loss

Guava flower essences, one cup of guava tea per day, hair-rinsing and massage, concentrated guava tea.

Other support: Symbiotic Colon therapy, workstations, head massages and Lymphatic drainage, Reflex zone massage, vitamin H, vitamin B. Washings with Aloe and yarrow infusion.

Homeopathic: Silicea D12, Sulphur D6.

Heart, Nervous Disturbances

Guava tincture is added to the bath water. Homeopathic Guava D12.

Other support: St. John's Wort, hawthorn, Cactus D12, therapeutic exercise, relaxation therapy

Headaches

The foreheads and temples are rubbed with crushed leaves. Alternatively guava leaf tea (including the leaves) is taken. Guava vinegar is added to the water.

Other support: Compresses in the neck with lavender oil, massage with lemon balm oil at the temples, acupuncture, Symbiotic Colon therapy, decontamination, Neural-therapy, relaxation therapy, Rosemary or basil in essential oil burner.

Hemorrhoids and Perianal Eczema

500gm fresh and 250gm dried fruit is mixed with water and boiled (stirred) until it becomes a thick mass. The inflamed area is treated repeatedly with this pulp.

Other support: Calendula oil, Senna leaves, papaya diet, Alder bark, Symbiotic Colon therapy, change of diet.

Immune System-Strengthening

Regularly are 3 fresh fruit consumed daily. Alternatively guava leaf tea is taken.

Other support: urine therapy, autohomological blood therapy, therapeutic exercise, relaxation therapy.

Intestinal Infections (Colitis)

Weak tea from young leaves, homeopathic Guava D6, *nux vomica*.

Other support: Diet, Symbiotic Colon therapy, ear acupuncture.

Impetigo

Combine 100ml of a decoction of guava to which you add 10 drops of lavender essential oil, using cotton wool wash the sores out thoroughly. Then make up a compress to which you add essential oils of tagets and myrrh to a decoction of guava and apply to sores.

Itching
Soak into a guava bath to which you add ½ cup of guava vinegar, ½ cup of fine oatmeal and 6 drops of a combination of lavender and chamomile essential oil. Use guava lotion on its own or add chamomile essential oil to lotion. Apply to affected areas 2–3 times a day for relief.

Kidney Infection and Kidney Colic
See also urinary tract infection.

Very weak guava tea is taking in large quantities.

Menstruation, Pains
A strong tea is cooked from the young shoots (with leaf) and repeatedly taken several times a day.

Other support: Agnus cactus, Silverweed, Cimicifuga, acupuncture, reflexzone massage

Mucus Membranes—Irritation
Cook a handful of leaves (alternatively 2 teaspoons of dried leaf powder) for 5 minutes. After cooling down, it is used for rinsing the mouth or as vaginal douche.

Other support: added tinctures from Arnica, Calendula or Hamamelis are beneficial for healing.

Change of diet, Symbiotic Colon therapy.

Obesity

Guava fruit juice diluted with plenty of water is taken repeatedly, for better results Artichokes and Dandelion are added. Alternatively 3–4 weak guava tea is taken

Other support: adjustment of diet, therapeutic exercise, relaxation therapy, homeopathic detoxification, ear acupuncture, Kneipp therapy.

Pain—Guava for Pain Relief

Treatments can help conditions such as various forms of joint pain arthritis, gout and muscular pain as rheumatism and fibrosis.

Compresses may be used for therapeutic applications. They can help to relieve pain, swelling and inflammation. Hot compresses are generally used to relieve chronic pain, while cold compresses are used for acute pain. To alternate hot and cold compresses are very beneficial.

Pain Relief Compresses

Guava Vinegar 50ml
Hot water 450ml
Juniper essential oil 10 drops
Chamomile essential oil 10 drops
Rosemary essential oil 5 drops

Agitate the essential oils with other ingredients then add a cloth to mixture wring out and apply to affected area.

Pain Relief Bath

Guava vinegar ½ cup
Guava oil 5ml
Juniper 4 drops
Cypress 2 drops
Marjoram Essential oil 2 drops
Lavender essential oil 2 drops

This bath is also excellent for rheumatism and general aches and pain. The recommended bathing time is 10–15 minutes.

To avoid evaporation of the essential oils in the mixtures it is recommended to add the oils to the bath water after filling the tub.

Pain Relief Oil

Guava oil 20ml
Virgin olive oil 10ml
Chamomile 10 drops
Marjoram 10 drops
Lavender 5 drops
Rosemary 5 drops

Mix ingredients together and massage in to affected areas when needed. For best results use oil after guava compresses or a bath.

Pancreas Disorders
Guava fruits as a major part of diet, large quantities of, with clear water diluted, guava and other fruit juices

Other support: diet: Tea fasting or if necessary pineapple and/or papaya diet, melons, Symbiotic Colon therapy

Psoriasis
Make up a skin wash with a combination of a decoction of guava leaves mixed with turmeric, wash affected area before applying the oil blend.

Psoriasis Oil Mixture

> Guava oil 40ml
> Papaya oil 40ml
> Castor oil 20ml
> add essential oils of Bergamot 25 drops
> Chamomile 10 drops
> Yarrow 5 drops
> Carrot seed 5 drops
> Lavender 5 drops

Mix well and apply to affected areas twice a day.

Rheumatism, see pains
Rubbings (3 or 4 times daily) onto the affected joints with the inside of the bark, or with guava lotion. Guava tea 3-4 cups guava tea is taken daily, 2-3 fresh fruit are

eaten daily. Guava-Kombucha fungus compresses. See also Arthrose.

Scalds and Burns
Use dried fruit and heat till it turns charcoal. Then grind to powder add to rape oil and blend to a paste and apply to affected area.

Lavender essential oil can be used to help reduce pain, and promote rapid healing and will help to reduce scarring.

Scabies is a distressing condition, with intense itching, caused by a minute insect, the itch mite (sarcoptes scabei).

Treatment wash affected areas with a decoction of guava leaves, essential oils bergamot, lavender, peppermint, rosemary or tea tree can be added.

Scabies Lotion

Guava oil 50ml
Guava vinegar 50ml
Garlic capsules 2
add essential oils of Lavender 20 drops
Tea Tree 20 drops
Cinnamon 5 drops
Clove 5 drops

Combine and apply twice a day after washing affected areas with a decoction of guava.

Stomach Troubles generally
Guava bark or leaves are boiled and the infusion taken, dried fruits are eaten.

Other support: compresses with concentrated guava tea or guava tincture, massages of the stomach area with guava oil or ointment, Wormwood, Camomile, Fennel. Homeopathic *nux vomica*.

Throat Disorders
Gargling with cool guava leaf tea, ripe guava fruit flesh which is rich on vitamins especially vitamin C.

Other support: gargling with tea tree oil, sage or camomile.

Ulcers externally and internally see under skin diseases.

Urinary Tract Infections
Guava tea powder is briefly boiled and left to settle for at least 10 minutes. 3–4 litres are taken during the day. Guava juice diluted clear water is taken.

Other support: 3–6 cups of a herb tea mixture to equal parts Prostawort, Calendula and Horsetail is taken.

Worms
A handful of guava seeds is crushed mixed with honey and taken with warm water. This is repeated over 4–5 days. Papaya seeds are more efficient for all worms but should not be taken during pregnancy.

Symbiotic Colon therapy, water drinking regimen, *lactulosis* therapy.

Wounds
Wash affected area with a decoction of guava leaves and apply fresh crushed fruit to the affected area, repeat twice a day.

Essential oils of lavender, tea tree or myrrh is useful for any wounds that are slow to heal.

Toothache
The inner bark of the tree is chewed against toothache. Fresh leaves can be chewed as well. In the Philippines the leaves are squeezed first and than placed to the affected area in the mouth.

Vomiting
In the Philippines inhalations are used to settle the stomach, prepared from the young crushed shoots (with leaves).

Other support: *nux vomica*, acupuncture, camomile.

Does Guava Have Negative Side Effects?

The recommendations in the book are based on observations, experiences through history up to our present day and from modern scientific studies which have to be done over a longer period to give a clear answer if there is a possibility of undesirable side effects. Using guava in high dosages or concentrated form, as well as any other medicine or treatment, is at the individual's own risk. However, no negative side effects, including addiction, are known. As it is with all other remedies, including food, an intake in too large quantities and over a long period of time is not recommended. In the book *Juice—Diet for Perfect Health* it is mentioned by the Chinese authors (Dr Gala et. al) that large quantities of guava fruit should not be eaten and that people suffering from constipation should not eat the fruit (seeds). On the other hand the seeds are chewed in Malaysia against constipation.

Guava for Health and Beauty

Guava fruit and leaves can be used for health and beauty.

The guava fruit and leaves contain tannins which are utilised in cosmetics for a pronounced astringent effect, caused by their reaction with skin proteins. Under the influence of tannins a protective membrane is formed on damaged skin, the nerve endings are desensitised, the discharge of secretions is stopped and inflammations as well as irritation and itching are reduced.

Guava Skin Care

Guava fruit and leaves can be used in treating acne or blemished skin.

Skin Cleanser

>Pure Honey 50gm
>Guava Vinegar 5ml
>Lemon juice ml 1ml

Mix ingredients together. Apply twice daily onto moist skin and massage in gently, then rinse well with water.

Skin Toner

>Guava vinegar 20ml
>Lavender water 60ml

Mix ingredients together. Use twice daily after you have cleansed the skin.

Moisturising Oil

>Guava oil 20ml
>Yarrow oil 10ml
>Almond oil 15ml
>Evening primrose oil 5ml
>Carrot Seed Oil 5 drops
>Lavender Essential oil 10 drops

Mix ingredients together. Massage a few drops gently into the skin gently twice daily.

Face Mask

> Green clay 10gm
> Brewers yeast 5gm
> Guava powder 10gm

Mix ingredients together and add water until a soft paste. Apply with a soft brush. Avoid contact with the eyes! Let mask dry. Rinse with tepid water, following with guava skin toner and moisturising oil.

Use once a week.

Fresh Guava Facemask

> Guava fruit ¼
> Pure honey 1 teaspoon
> Egg whole 1
> Guava vinegar ¼ teaspoon
> Buttermilk 2 tablespoons

Mix ingredients together and apply to well cleansed skin. Leave for 10 to 15 minutes. Rinse with tepid water, then splash on Guava skin toner and apply a few drops Guava moisturising oil.

Spot Mix

> Guava oil 5ml
> Castor oil 5ml
> Guava vinegar 10ml

Tea tree essential oil 10 drops.

Shake mixture well before every use. Dab a small amount of spot mix onto troubled areas twice a day and in the evening until the spots has cleared. Use little to achieve maximum results.

Pimples and boils-grind the fresh guava leaves to a pulp and apply to spots or boils leave on for 15 minutes, rinse then and apply spot mix.

Guava Body Care

Guava used in body care and can assist in deodorising the body, eliminating dead skin cells and relieving itching skin.

Aromatic Bath

Guava vinegar ½ cup
Guava oil 5ml
Epsom salts
Lavender essential oil 5 drops
Bergamot essential oil 3 drops
Cypress essential oil 2 drops
Optional add ½ cup of fine oatmeal
for itchy skin conditions.

Bath once a week to relax, nourish and deodorise the skin.

Body Lotion

>Guava oil 20ml
>Guava vinegar 30ml
>Lavender essential oil 10 drops
>Bergamot 10 drops
>Cypress 5 drops

Shake all ingredients together before applying to the body, for best results use after aromatic bath to deodorise the body.

Body Powder

>Guava powder 50g
>Arrowroot 50g
>Lavender essential oil 20 drops
>Bergamot essential oil 15 drops
>Lemon grass essential oil 15 drops.

Add essential oils to dry ingredients into a glass container and close the lid, leave overnight then place through a flour sieve. Keep in a sealed container and use as a deodorising powder.

Body Rub

Ground guava leaves to a paste and mix with fine oatmeal, sea salt and water then apply all over the body for a smoother deodorised body. Then soak in an aromatic bath for 15 minutes.

Under Arm Deodorant

>Guava vinegar 50ml
>Witch hazel 50ml
>Lavender 25 drops
>Lemongrass 15 drops
>Cypress essential oil 10 drops

Add essential oils to guava vinegar leave in a sealed bottle over night. Strain through a filter then add witch hazel. Keep in an atomiser and spray on as a natural deodorant.

Hair Care

Guava bark and leaves can be used in shampoo and as a hair rinse for shining hair and to relieve itchy scalp conditions.

Hair Pre-Conditioner

>Guava oil 10ml
>Guava vinegar 5ml
>Whole egg 1
>Rosemary essential oil 5 drops

Shake lotion and apply to dry hair, wrap hair into a towel and leave on for 10 minutes.

Apply shampoo straight onto hair conditioner before adding water, shampoo twice and rinse well. To the final rinse add 2 tablespoons of guava vinegar.

Hair Shampoo

Castle liquid soap 5ml
Guava vinegar 1ml
Distilled water 5ml
Rosemary essential oil 3 drops
Sandalwood essential oil 2 drops

Mix well and wash hair with shampoo, can be used for normal hair and to relieve an itchy scalp.

Hair Rinse

Guava vinegar 2 tablespoons
Rosemary essential oil 2 drops
Sandalwood essential oil 2 drops

Add to the final rinse water for a healthier scalp.

Hair Lotion

Boil up guava leaves and old bark allow to cool. Rub into scalp and hair for healthier shiny hair.

Head Lice

Guava leaves boiled up to a thick liquid mixed with turmeric can be applied for head lice. As a prevention essential oils of rosemary, geranium, lavender, eucalyptus and lemon are a lice deterrent. Add 2 drops of any of the essential oils to 1 tablespoon of guava vinegar to the final hair rinse.

Guava Foot Care

Guava can be used as a natural deodoriser. Soaking the feet in guava footbath can assist in eliminating foot odour.

Foot Odour is caused by wearing synthetic footwear: socks, stockings and tights. The usual advice is to wear natural fibre shoes to let the skin breathes; cotton or woollen socks.

Treatment: Regular use of guava in footbaths and by applying guava foot lotion and powder can assist to regulate foot odour and perspiration.

Footbath

Guava Vinegar 20ml
Epsom salt 25g
Tea tree Essential oils 2 drops
Sage essential oil 2 drops
Lavender essential oil 2 drops

Agitate essential oils to a bowl of hot water large enough to place your feet into, then add guava vinegar. Soak feet for a minimum of 10 to 15 minutes at least twice a week.

Foot Lotion

>Guava vinegar 50ml
>Witch hazel 30ml
>Distilled water 20ml
>Cypress 20 drops
>Lavender 20 drops
>Peppermint 10 drops

Mix essential oils in guava vinegar, Leave over night, strain through a filter, add remaining ingredients. Shake well and apply daily for maximum benefit use after a footbath.

Foot Powder

>Guava powder 2 tablespoons
>Cornstarch 1 tablespoon
>Sage essential oil 4 drops
>Lavender essential oil 2 drops

Blend ingredients together and dust feet with powder and leave ½ teaspoon in shoes over night.

Other Uses of Guava

Wood for Smoking for the Barbecue
Guava wood has a sweetish aroma and is used for barbecuing and for smoking of fish, lamb, pork, chicken and beef. It gives the food a very pleasant taste. In Hawaii and India guava wood is a available to the trade. Charcoal from guava has been produced in Hawaii since the turn of the century.

Tanning of Leather
The leaves have with 9% to 11% a high content of tannin. Also the bark is rich in tannin. Guava tannin the most popular tannin for most purposes is widely used in India. Manufacturers of shoes prefer leather manufactured with guava tannin, since the leather is smooth and doesn't crack as leathers manufactured with other tannins.

Wood Processing
In the homeland of the guava, the red Indians made their spears from Guava wood. It is still used today for woodcarvings. The grey-brown wood, with its typical proportionate fibre, also suits wood turning very well.

In India, which is nowadays the most important country in guava production, instruments are manufactured from Guava wood.

Dyeing

In India the leaves are used to dye silk. The production process for the dye, the *"ayer banyar"*, takes 3–4 months. Fresh guava leaves are mixed with some other plant parts, all containing tannin, with Coconut milk and some iron is added. In China a liquid is manufactured from guava, which dyes cotton black.

Washing After Burial

In the Philippines it is a custom that one washes the hands after a burial in a tea made from guava and other herbs.

Dental Hygiene

Young guava branches are used to make a simple toothbrush.

Practical Hints for Better Health and Vigour

1. Exercise
- Daily in the morning 10 minutes gymnastics.
- The Five Tibetan Rites by the open window.
- In the evening 30 minutes sport or an hour walk.

2. Nourishment
- Whole grain bread, musli, milk (unprocessed), yoghurt, fresh fruit, vegetables and salads as daily basic food.

- Drinking of 2 to 3 litre per day.
- No meat or sausage, except a maximum of once a week.
- Never eat without hunger or in a hurry.
- Eat slowly and chew well.

3. Natural Factors
- Hardening through cold shower, sauna, fresh air, sun.
- Regular sleep a minimum of 7 hours beginning before midnight.

4. Your Time
- Do not "waste" time.
- Utilise your time for learning and further development or to rejuvenate body and mind, doing things which make you happy and amuse you. Things you really like for sufficient regular sleep care

5. Relaxation Training
- Regular meditation (20 minutes daily) or autogenic training, best immediately after stretching gymnastics and the Five Tibetan Rites.

The Time will come...

"The time will come, when the task of a doctor will not be to treat the body but to heal the mind, which in turn will heal the body.

*In other words, the right doctor will be philosopher and teacher
and it will be his concern to keep the person healthy
and not to start treating the body when it has already become sick.
The true doctor will not only treat the body with medication,
but rather treat the mind with principles.
He will teach people that good humour, goodwill, noble deeds,
love and grace are just as beneficial for the body as for the mind
and that a joyous heart is the best medicine.
Positive, pure thoughts are the premise for purity of the body,
for inner harmony and balanced serenity."*

Waldo Trine (American philosopher, 1899)

The Way to Freedom

Clean up inwardly. Create order within yourself, peace and quietness, so that an intense feeling of freedom and tranquillity can establish itself.

Live the feeling of the moment, which is the only time, in which life really occurs—here and now. If you are able to live the moment in its full beauty attentively and intensely, your life gains in a multiple of ways in colour and beauty.

1. Create internal harmony through meditation or just time, which belongs only to you.

2. Find out what you really want. Formulate your dreams and goals and pray that they come true. If someone has no goals they cannot achieve any.

3. Think positive in all situations and be generous with positive thoughts toward persons who need them.

4. Do several good deeds every day and meet all the other people with love and goodness. "There is nothing good, unless one does it".

5. Always keep this point in your mind: the quality of your thoughts determines the quality of your daily life experiences.

6. Listen and trust the voice of your intuition, she will point you the right way in all difficult situations. Only give your intuition the chance to talk to you for example during meditation.

7. Act in all things so that you can answer for each of your deeds before yourself and before others.

8. Do only things to others which you wish that they do to you.

9. Live end love.

Final Remark from Harald

Like with all good medicinal plants or remedies, it is only a question of time, until someone finds negative effects (true or not true) in very old remedies. They are then suddenly rated as threatening poison. Hawthorn, Compfrey, Kombucha, St. Benedict and many other medicinal herbs and foods were outlawed in the past in some countries and then became legal again.

With "new" discovered traditional remedies it happens, that enemies of the remedy, predominantly propelled by the chemical industry, campaign against the remedy. Since there is not only very limited money in traditional medicine, it is extremely hard to defend indications against time-honoured proven healing remedies.

We have to start to learn to think for ourselves and have to ask our own internal voice what is good or harmful for us. For many years, after I had written my first book about Earthrays, I have given innumerable seminars to show people how to discover and to develop their sixth sense. If someone takes a remedy, natural or chemical alike, they should ask the internal voice, whether it is good for the individual or not. In the same way, each sensitive person who developed their natural sense can find out for themselves how much one can take or should take and over what period of time. A new remedy always works better than a remedy which is taken over a longer period of time. The body must be stimulated again and again or there must be a break in a treatment with an alternative treatment to stimulate the body continuously. This is the case for mixtures of remedies, which must be altered likewise from time to time for best results.

We are all individuals and react differently to different remedies. A remedy which helps one person, can be dangerous for another person. The easiest example to explain this is tea. A person with very low blood pressure who drinks some cups of coffee or tea (greens tea, black tea, Mate tea) everyday can feel excellent. The caffeine in these drinks gives the necessary increase of blood pressure and with it better feeling. A person with a too high blood pressure on the other hand can feel uncomfortable and the stimulation could even trigger serious conditions.

Besides the green and black tea there is the semi-fermented oolong tea. The source of all these common teas on the market is the tea bush (*Camellia sinensis*). The teas known as English breakfast teas, Russian teas, etc. are black teas (fermented teas). Many of the fermented teas are also blended with other teas e.g. with Bergamot or other substances like lavender oil which gives the "Earl Grey" its flavour. Most people in the Western world drink common black or oolong tea instead of green tea probably because of the stronger flavour.

Many individuals feel a fast stimulating effect when drinking black tea, the same as that experienced when drinking coffee. For this reason, people who suffer from an irritable bladder favour tea over coffee. Green tea, on the other hand, does not stimulate as rapidly or as highly as black tea and coffee, but has a steadier and longer lasting effect. The alkaloid caffeine (between 1% and 5% in tea) is responsible for the stimulating effect of tea.

Caffeine stimulates the central nervous system as well as the action of the lungs and the heart. It also promotes urine production. Caffeine is not only in common teas like black, green, and oolong tea which are all from the same plant—the tea bush (*Camellia sinensis*), but also in coffee (*Coffea arabica*), cola drinks from the cola nut (*Cola nitida* and *C. acuminata*) mate tea (ilex paraguariensis) and cacao in chocolate (*Theobroma cacao*).

In recent times green tea has frequently been mentioned as a potential anti-cancer aid. Dr Robert E. Willner (USA), author of the book *The Cancer Solution* mentions the 'delicate pale tea' as a source of anti-carcinogenic substances. Green tea contains the chemical "Epigallocatechin Gallate" (EGCG) which inhibits the growth of cancer and lowers the cholesterol levels. *"Green tea gives health and longevity"* is an old Buddhist saying.

The Japanese go further in utilising the healing benefits of green tea—the tea leaves are eaten, as with normal tea consumption (as a drink) a considerable portion of the precious vitamins and trace elements are thrown away. Professor Kazutami Kuwano of the Kasei Gakuin Junior College (Chikaro Shimoaka *Green tea—more than a health drink*) closely investigated the "tea-food". He came to the conclusion that the high content of vitamin A and E that is contained in green tea, is not accessible to the body since these vitamins are not water-soluble. Calcium, iron and vitamin C in the tea beverage are only half utilised compared to when it is eaten. For 3 cups of green tea one uses approximately 6gm of tea leaves—a teaspoonful. This quantity of tea when eaten contains 50% of our daily vitamin E, and 20% of our vitamin A requirements and there are virtually no calories in tea leaves.

The healing effect of green tea depends on the quality of the product. The quality of the tea differs according to where the tea is grown, the harvest (whether vital young leaves or old leaves) and the processing procedures.

Quality losses due to storage conditions and storage time have to be taken into consideration. This also applies to every other medicinal herb.

What has all this to do with guava? Quite a lot, since medicinal guava teas are made from the leaves, the bark and even from the roots, they are successfully used against many diseases. The guava leaf tea can be brewed like ordinary tea. As we have learnt from the ordinary tea, it is however more advisable for medicinal purposes, to consume the tea leaves (powder) with the tea liquid. In this way all valuable ingredients of the tea are utilised and not flushed down in the kitchen sink.

We hope that you find help with our story about this extraordinary medicinal plant. Perhaps guava will give you, like many other people before, health and new vigour.

Bibliography

Aihara, Herman. *Acid & Alkaline*, George Ohsawa Macrobiotic Foundation, Oroville, USA, 1986.

Bakhru, H.K. *Foods that Heal: The Natural Way to Good Health*, Orient Paperbacks, Delhi, India, 1996.

Chaitow, Leon. *Probiotics: the revolutionary "friendly bacteria" way to vital health and well-being*, Thorsons Publishers Limited, Wellingborough, England, 1990.

Cilento, R. Dr. *Heal Cancer*, Hill of Content, Melbourne, Australia, 1993.

Eliot, R. & De Paoli, C. *Kitchen Pharmacy*, Tiger Books International, London, England, 1994.

Foster, Ted. *Pawpaw growing*, Division of Agricultural Services, NSW, Australia, 1991.

Grieve, M. *A Modern Herbal*, Tiger Books International, London, England, 1994.

Gurudas. *Flower Essences and Vibrational Healing*, Brotherhood of Life, New Mexico, USA, 1987.

Gurudas. *The Spiritual Properties of Herbs*, Cassandra Press, San Rafael, California, USA. 1988.

Hobert, Ingfried, M.D. *Heilungsgeheimnisse der Aborigines*, Peter Erd Verlag München 1998.

Hobert, Ingfried, M.D. *Das Heilbuch für das neue Jahrtausend*, Peter Erd Verlag, München 1997.

Hobert, Ingfried, M.D. *Gesundheit selbst gestalten—Wege der Selbstheilung und die "Fünf Tibeter"* Integral Verlag, Wessobrunn 1993.

Hobert, Ingfried, M.D. *Handbuch der natürlichen Medizin*, Ariston Verlag Genf 1997.

Klock, Peter. *Früchte, Gemüse und Gewürze aus dem Süden*, BLV München, 1990.

Lötschert, Wilhelm. *Pflanzen der Tropen*, BLV München, 1992.

Low, Tim. *Bush Medicine* Harper Collins Publishers, London, 1990.

Lucas, R. *Nature's Medicines*, First Award Printing, New York, USA, 1974.

Newsletter "Health for all" Tietze Publishing, P.O. Box 34 Bermagui 2546, Pedersen,Mark, *Nutritional Herbology, A Reference Guide, to Herbs,* Wendell W. Whitman Company, Warsaw, USA, 1992.

Padua de, Ludivina, Gregorio Lugod, Juan Pancho. *Handbook on Philippine Medicinal Plants,* University of the Philippines at Los Banos.

Popenoe, Wilson. *Manual of tropical and subtropical fruits,* The Macmillan Company, New York, USA, 1974.

Readers Digest, "Magic in Medicine of Plants", Surry Hills, Australia, 1994.

Rose, J. *Herbs & Things,* Putnam Publishing Group, New York, 1983.

Saha, N.N. *Fruit and Vegetable Juice Therapy,* B. Jain Publishers New Delhi, India, 1996.

Schultes, Richard & Robert Raffauf. *The Healing Forest.*

Tankard, G.J. *Rare and exotic tree fruit for the Australian home garden,* Thomas Nelson, Victoria, Australia, 1987.

Tietze, W.H. *Herbal Teaology,* P.O. Box 34 Bermagui 2546, Australia, 1996.

Tietze, W.H. *Kombucha, Gesund & Fit mit dem Wunderpilz,* mvg-Verlag, Landsberg am Lech, Germany, 1996.

Tietze, W.H. *Shivambu, Urin-das heilige Wasser,* mvg-Verlag, Landsberg am Lech, Germany, 1997.

Tietze, W.H. *Spirulina, Micro Food—Macro Blessings,* PHREE Books, P.O. Box 34 Bermagui 2546, Australia, 1996.

Trenorden, Jan. *The Essences and Chironic Healing*, PHREE Books, P.O. Box 34 Bermagui 2546, Australia.

Zinßfang, Dai & Lui Cheng-jun. *Yao Yong Guo Pin* The Rams Skull Press, Kurunda, Australia, 1986.

References

"Identification of gallocatechin as a bio-antimutagenic compound in Psidium guava leaves" *Phytochemistry* 36 (1994) 1027–9.

"Can Guava fruit intake decrease blood pressure and blood lipids" *Journal of Human Hypertension* 7 (1993) 33–38.

"Effects of guava intake on serum total and high density lipoprotein cholesterol levels and on systemic blood pressure." *American Journal of Cardiology* 70 (1992) 1287–91.

"Physical chemical characteristics of partially clarified guava juice and concentrate" *Journal of Food Science* 55 (1990) 1757–8.

"Studies on the Physio-chemical composition of fruits of twenty guava varieties." *Indian Food Packer* 49 (1995) 15–35.

"Biochemical and physical changes in fruits of four guava cultivars during growth and development" *Food Chemistry* 54 (1995) 279.

"Quercetin Glycosides in *Psidium guajava*" *Archives of Medical Research* 25 (1994) 11–.

"Calcium Antagonist effect of Quercetin and its relation with the spasmolytic properties of *psidium guajava*" *AMR* 25 (1994) 17–.

"Antidiarrhoel activity of the methanolic fraction of the extract of unripe fruits of *Psidium guajava*" *Phytotherapy Research* 7 (1993) 431–.

"Analgetic efficacy of *Psidium guajava* extractive in mouse experimental pain models" *Asia Pacific Journal of Pharmacology* 8 (1993) 83–.

"Inhibition of microlax induced experimental diarrhoea with narcotic like extracts of psidium guajava leaves" *Journal of Ethnopharmacology* 37 (1992) 151–.

"Hypoglycemic effect of Guava juice in mice and human subjects" *American Journal of Chinese Medicine* 11 (1983) 74–76.

"Quercetin a Bioflavonoid inhibits the induction of interleukin 8 and monocyte chemoattractant protein 1 expression by Tumour necrosis factor a in cultured human synovial cells" *Journal of Rheumatology* 24 (1997) 1680–.

"Quercetin enhances transforming growth factor b1 secretion by human ovarian cancer cells" *International Journal of Cancer* 57 (1994) 211–215.

"Quercetin mediates the down regulation of mutant p53 in the human breast cancer cell line" *Cancer Research* 54 (1994) 2424–.